Mother's Intention
How Belief Shapes Birth

Revised and updated-2nd edition

By Kim Wildner

Intuitu LLC, 2012

Disclaimer:

This book has been written in the attempt to help women make their own best choices regarding their births. The whole point of the book is for women to research their options and initiate dialog with their care providers about their options. No action should be taken without consultation with a qualified health care professional. Mother's Intention is not meant to replace the advice of any health care professional.

Persons following any course of action as a result of this book do so of their own free will and do not hold the author or publisher responsible for any problems encountered as a result of said action. The reader assumes all responsibility for their own health and care during their pregnancy, birth and postpartum period.

Do not use as a substitute for childbirth education classes, but as an enhancement. Great effort has been made to assure compatibility with all independent classes centered on evidence-based care and informed consumerism.

Personal accounts are either composites of many situations with identifying core material altered, or the parties involved have given permission for inclusion. Any resemblance to people, living or deceased, is purely coincidental.

First edition released September, 2003
Second edition released September, 2012
Intuitu, LLC, Wisconsin, USA
www.kimwildner.me
Cover Photography by Chelsea Wildner

What people are saying about this revolutionary work:

"In *Mother's Intention* Wildner has given to all women who are pregnant and to all who wish to be pregnant an honest, accurate and clearly marked roadmap for their journey toward achieving safe and comfortable birthing. It is a must read!"
Marie F. Mongan, Founder HypnoBirthing® Institute
www.hypnobirthing.com

"If everyone were to read this book and honestly venture into their own beliefs regarding pregnancy, birth and parenthood, great things would happen! Our country's infant mortality rate would drastically decline, women would fully embrace the power of their femininity, and best of all, the act of birth would no longer be feared. It would be anticipated with joy, engaged in totally, and treasured as the miracle it is!"
Lynette M. Prentice A.A.H.C.C.
Birth Instructor and Mother of three

"This book provides pregnant families with an opportunity to explore their beliefs and feelings around pregnancy and birth. Opportunities for contemplation and journaling thread throughout the book, helping families clarify their own thoughts and feelings with a fresh perspective."
Pat Sonnenstuhl, CNM, HBCE, CPPI

"It's time to quit the whining, and take our births back. No more "I didn't know", "Where were you when I had my baby", "Nobody told me". Here it is. It IS possible for birth to be a peak experience, and it's worth working for. Ms. Wildner provides both theory and tools to help women shape this amazing event. So read the book, do the thinking, and create the framework for the experience you want for yourself, your baby and your life."
Kip Kozlowski, RN, CNM, CHt.
Director, Greenhouse Birth Center

Dedication:

This work is dedicated to my loving husband, Dave, whose unwavering faith made this book possible and to my gorgeous daughter, Chelsea Raine, whose gentle birth inspired me to use my life toward improving the world she will inherit. I love you both.

I am also grateful for the many parents who have expanded my horizons. I've learned innumerable lessons from their joy...and pain. I would specifically like to thank Shelley and Alan for believing in me more than I believed in myself, and Rebecca for showing me how strong women really are.

To the many professionals within the birthing community, working diligently for better birth, I thank you. My own 'fairytale' birth, possible through the efforts of those who have ceaselessly poured their hearts into improving birth outcomes for the last 30 or more years, empowered me. My paradigm shift regarding pain and birth could not have happened without Mickey Mongan. My introduction to HypnoBirthing® planted the seed that became a garden.

I'd like to thank Yolanda Visser, for first suggesting that maybe the Universe was trying to steer me toward writing and education.

Trish Telsesco also suggested I collect my thoughts and share them. I didn't listen to her at first either! I am grateful for those that kept trying to point out my strengths and helped me refine them.

My best friend Diane lifted me through frustrations and shared my epiphanies at all hours of the day and night, all while nursing two boys through babyhood. I am grateful for her stamina and the unique ability she has to nourish my soul.

I would like to thank Kip Koslowski for helping me sort out my thoughts; for her seemingly endless reservoir of support and encouragement as well as her wit and expertise. Without her help this work truly would never have come to fruition. Her wisdom kept me in line. Her humor kept me laughing, and her affection kept my spirits up.

And finally everyone who supported the first edition of this work!

Contents

Foreword, 2003

We have this saying in the doula world; "Knowledge is power." The most important thing you can do for yourself and your baby is to take away all the misinformation provided by friends and family. All you tend to hear are horror stories everywhere you turn. I feel that this happens because they didn't feel like they had the right to question or dream of that beautiful birth.

Well, beautiful births happen all the time and I know this because I am at those births with my clients. They come in all different ways. Some of my clients use midwives but most of them are in a hospital and they choose a place and a doctor that have the same belief system and are open to what the mom feels is the right way for her and her baby to deliver. It really comes down to what you feel is right for you.

Kim has written a book that I call a map to your birth. When you are going to take a trip in a car somewhere, you pull out a map and you look for all the ways to get there.

Let's say you are going to grandma's house and you haven't been there since you were a kid. Grandma hasn't left her house in years. You call her and she starts telling you how to get there. She tells you that it will take about 10 hours. She then starts telling you that you will need to bring chains for your tires because the snow can be really deep at the pass. She also tells you that you need to bring extra gas because if the snow is too deep the one gas station might be closed. You say goodbye to her and hang up the phone and you start thinking that there has got to be a better way there. So, you get your map and start looking and see that there are a lot of different ways to get to Grandma's house. There are roads that are completely paved and roads that go by beautiful streams and waterfalls. And you notice that on every road there are forks that you can take at any time to change your direction or length of your trip. You notice that you never have to go over that pass that causes so much of the problem. You feel relieved and so glad that there are maps to make this trip something to be excited about.

This book is YOUR map to your birth. It is a map of all the different ways to have your baby with all the information of every way so that you can take the road you want and when you have forks in the road you'll know which one to take because you'll know what each road and fork offers you and the outcomes it delivers.

Thank you Kim, for putting this in a form that all can understand. There are no agendas here. There is no shame here if you pick a birth that is not "natural."

This is a training book for many if not all things in your life. You will be changed after reading this book and on the road to a healthy and beautiful birth with no regrets or questions unanswered.

Dee Nipper, Doula and Executive producer and host of The Real Side of Birth, A positive radio show about birth and your choices

Dee's partner, Sheri Menelli says:

A few years ago, I began a journey to empower moms and dads during birth.

It started after several of the couples from my class went into a downward after a prenatal visit. Sometimes they were told that the baby was going to be too big, that they didn't have enough amniotic fluid, that the due date was changing again or that they couldn't have the birth they wanted for any number of other reasons.

I felt helpless. I wanted to help, but moms and dads could not get past the belief that birth was flawed. What I saw over, and over again, were moms who were completely panicked and fearful before the birth, and very angry after the birth.

Once in a while I would see a couple who would ask the provider question after question and do their own research until they were fully educated on the matter. If they met resistance from a care giver about having the birth their way, these clients would usually hunt for a new doctor who could meet their high expectations. They had fabulous births.

Some couples had providers who were verbally abusive before the birth. They did not bother to find a better care provider. During the birth the care provider was still abusive. The couple did not enjoy the birth of their baby and they had quite a bit of anger that lasted for months, if not years.

I prayed for a tool that could help them. I even started producing and co-hosting a radio show called "The Real Side of Birth" with the purpose of better educating the couples as early as possible. I didn't think it was possible that someone in another part of the country would not only feel the same way as I did but would find away of explaining so eloquently how these challenges could be resolved. When I read the book, *Mother's Intention*, I cried. My tears were of sadness for the many women who didn't have this resource before having their babies and tears of joy that I was privy to one of the most amazing books that I'd ever read. I was glued to the book for two days. I found the answers that I had been searching for. I finally had a resource that my clients could read that would change the course of their birth. This resource would guide them through the medical system. As I read each chapter, I was startled by all of the new information I learned about birthing. There were things I never thought about questioning before, that now were so obvious. I hope that this will be the first book that women will read when they discover that they are pregnant. I'm sure that you will find this book to be one of the most helpful of all guides in your journey to have a wonderful and happy birthing day.

Sheri Menelli Certified HypnoBirthing Educator and Certified Hypnotherapist Producer and Co-Host of The Real Side of Birth

Foreword to 2nd edition, 2012

A Note from the author:

Ten years ago I had a high school education, a passion to help mothers make decisions that would lead to safer, more comfortable birth (a couple of childbirth education certifications and an entry level midwifery education to back that up) and a pile of sticky notes full of wisdom from self-help gurus.

In my own journey of self-discovery, I had begun to notice that what resonated with me when I watched Dr. Phil or Oprah was really not new information. Toni Robbins and Wayne Dyer had been saying the same things for years, in different ways and with different audiences listening. Before that, there were certainly others. This was recycled information. If so many successful individuals were getting so many people to listen over decades, there must be something to it.

In my professional life, I knew that the intention of most mothers was pure in making pregnancy, birthing and parenting decisions. However, even with baby's best interest in mind, very often those decisions did not result in the desired outcomes. Often they *did* result in *predictable* outcomes.

I wondered what would happen if healthy pregnant couples asked themselves the same things that life coaches asked of their clients. I collected these bits of wisdom on these little pieces of paper and incorporated them into my personal exchanges and eventually my classes. I started to see those 'light bulb' moments happen in mothers more often. Mothers did begin to wonder at the rationale of certain routine interventions that were not supported by evidence. Yet, they were still choosing caregivers who insisted on those interventions. They still consented to those interventions. I wondered why the better understanding didn't translate into different behavior. I didn't know it at the time, but my curiosity would lead me into psychological, sociological, philosophical, anthropological and theological inquiry. I was developing a thesis: Mothers want the best for their babies. Mothers are making pregnancy, birthing and parenting decisions that evidence shows are at best not helpful and at worst potentially harmful. Why? The U.S. has some of the worst maternal and infant outcomes in the developed world. We know what makes birth safer in the countries with the best outcomes. (Wagner, 2000) Why are so few people aware of how U.S. outcomes compare with other countries? Why is it that even women who are aware make choices that are contrary to what they know could make their birth safer? Why do women not just consent to, but actively seek out, maternity care that is demonstrably inferior to those countries with the best outcomes? In the U.S. we have a birthing paradigm based on fear and dependence and consider it 'normal.' Why, when exposed to a different birthing reality, based on empowerment and safety, do so many women still reject it when it might result in an ecstatic birth and make parenting infinitely easier?

Since asking myself these questions I've come to understand some concepts that might explain, at least a little bit, why we do what we do when faced with ideas contrary to what we believe. One such concept is 'confirmation bias,' which allows us to see only that which supports our current thinking. This book is my attempt at trying to figure out how to help women have safer, more satisfying births by understanding but a few of the reasons we behave in the ways we do. The complexity of the issue will likely mean I'll likely spend my whole life trying to figure it out.

I sought out resources in order to find supporting evidence defending my newly forming thesis. In doing so, I realized that adult learners have different needs, and often those needs aren't met. I needed to understand how to convey my thoughts to adult learners in a way that they would be most likely to accept these new ideas and utilize them for their own highest good. This led me to resources on critical thinking skills and communication.

My sticky notes became articles. People read my articles and asked me to talk about my ideas. As an introvert from a small town, that was intimidating, but my passion for the topic was bigger than my fear. This just felt right. It felt like it would make a difference if I could reach the people who were ready to hear what I had to say.

I pulled the articles into chapters. In some of them, I had mentioned HypnoBirthing® so I sent those to Marie Mongan, founder of HypnoBirthing, for content approval. I was sending out query letters and even hand-bound copies of the manuscript to people I hoped would help me figure out what to do with this work that had rather developed a life of its own.

In spring of 2003 Marie informed me that if I completed and published the book by fall of that year (just 6 months away!) she would provide a venue to launch it at the HypnoBirthing conclave in New Hampshire. Though the task seemed daunting, I thought of one of my favorite quotes. Actress Tina Fey once said that the best advice she had ever received was, (and I'm paraphrasing here), 'Always say yes. Then figure out how to make it happen.' This was one of the first instances in which I realized what good advice that truly is. I said "Yes!" and only later worried about how I would do it.

I had no idea that what I was doing was the equivalent of an autodidactic college level business course. I sent the copies of the manuscript to friends who were doctors, nurses, midwives, and grammar geeks. I asked them to fit this 336 page work into their lives and give me feedback...in just weeks. In researching printers, I had discovered that in order to have an actual book in my hands by September, I had to have everything arranged and at the printers no later than June, and that was pushing it. In the meantime, I figured out how to obtain ISBN numbers, had to work out a marketing strategy, learn how to distribute my finished product and launch my new publishing house...all by the end of the summer.

Had I known what I was doing, I would not have done it. My cluelessness allowed me to keep taking on each new task. My husband's absolute belief in me kept me excited about the possibilities. He was in the midst of changing jobs that summer which meant he could cash out his retirement. It wasn't enough to retire on, but *was* just the right amount of capital needed to launch this project. In retrospect, without the foreknowledge of what the economy was going to do, that was pretty stupid of us. Romantic, but stupid. However, we were both certain that it would make a difference in the lives of mothers, babies and families, so we plodded on.

Long story short, we launch the book in September of 2003 in New Hampshire.

Indeed it did make a difference. By the following year someone had contacted me who said that it had changed the way she made parenting decisions, and she was so grateful. Childbirth educators, doctors and midwives carried copies in their lending libraries around the world, and it became required reading for one doula training course. Young women approached me at conferences with tears in their eyes, thanking me and asking me to sign their books. I got more and more invitations to speak, and discovered not only was I fairly decent at it, I liked it! I even coined the term Fearless Birthing™ and began teaching Fearless Birthing workshops about the country. I loved it!

I sold the entire first run, but between promotional costs and other business expenses, we had yet to recoup our expenses. Then the economy started to get weird. My husband's work situation become unstable, and it looked as if I'd have to get whatever job my high school education would get me to make ends meet; except there were no jobs were we lived. We moved.

By this time, I had decided that Fearless Birthing should actually be expanded into a college level, two semester, Woman's Studies course. As woman after woman told me, "I wish I'd know about this *before* I was pregnant (or pregnant the first time)!" it became obvious that reaching women when they were already pregnant was too late. I developed a curriculum outline based on my years of experience and my new discoveries. However, actually doing the work of a doctorate means little without the piece of paper. I went back to school to begin the journey to earn that paper cred.

I was actually okay with that, though. Not all feedback was positive on my book and I agreed with some of the criticism. I didn't write well. I wrote the way I spoke; sometimes, that was pretty blunt. I had incorporated so much of the self-help techniques I had been using that the line between I couldn't even always say where I had heard much of it to provide attribution. The book was riddled with spelling and grammatical errors. After all, I only gave my crack team of friends a couple of weeks to give me feedback. I didn't know how to cite my work or the proper way to provide attribution. I wanted to learn how to do all of that correctly. I needed more exposure to all those disciplines I was using to construct my theories.

I earned a BA in Communications from Marian University, graduating Magna Cum Laude, enjoying a validating moment when one of my professors, upon review of my extensive portfolio and without prompting by me, commented that this body of work was closer to the equivalent of a doctorate, not the baccalaureate I'd receive.

Exposure through more psychology, sociology, philosophy and anthropology have convinced me my thesis is tenable. The process by which we make our childbearing decisions is complex, but there is a way for women to take back their births. In order to make the safest decisions for ourselves and our children, we need to be able to make these decisions based on evidence, which we cannot evaluate if we can't get beyond the true reasons we make decisions inappropriate to our personal circumstance. The entire childbearing year *matters*, not just for the health of the child and the mother, but for the family and society as well.

Therefore women deserve to know the consequences of the choices they make when they are making decisions on behalf of their children!

I hoped that earning this degree would progress to the opportunity to earn the Master's that would allow me to teach. So far that hasn't happened. My heart is with this work, but I live in a world where this can only be my part-time obsession. I have not been offered the dream job of studying and teaching that will allow me to reach women earlier in their childbearing years, nor do I have a long-lost philanthropic relative, burning to make a difference in the world, who wants to pay my bills.

So, here I am again. I have grown as a communicator, not to mention a lot has happened in the birthing world since *Mother's Intention* was released in 2003. Some things that I predicted then have come to pass. I've mellowed out a little at 46, with a wider array of life experiences. Motivational speakers all say that the difference between winners and losers is that winners never give up. I'm not giving up.

What is different about this edition?

This edition differs from the first in that the writing has been cleaned up, so to speak. I have the assistance of my incredibly intelligent adult daughter, who is not only one of the most talented writers I know, but is also the most honest critic. Also, with the different perspective allowed by time, I see the work with fresh eyes. Finally, the statistics and references have been updated.

How to use this book

Essentially in order to have a safer, gentler, more empowering and emotionally satisfying birth (i.e. 'better' than you might otherwise have had, not 'better' in the sense that one way of birthing is superior to another) there is a linear progression of occurrences that

16

must take place. Thus, it is important to read the book sequentially.

PART ONE-INSPIRATION

First, there must be a realization that birth does not have to be the way it is portrayed in the media or the way many (if not most) women describe it. Certainly it can be. Certainly it has been. That does not mean it MUST be. But before any woman can have a different experience of it, she must simply be exposed to the idea that birth *can* be comfortable *and* safe. This sounds simple, but it is amazing how complex it really is. There are a multitude of reasons that women reject this idea. These are explored in Part One.

PART TWO-MOTIVATION

Just being exposed to the concept of a different view of birth doesn't magically transform birth, for an individual or collectively. So, why not? What makes birth safe? What causes discomfort in birth? How do our choices, from the beginning of pregnancy contribute to, or contaminate, the experience? This requires a high level of dedication to childbirth education (or re-education) and self-accountability. Birth is not something someone does for us. No one else except you and your baby will live with the consequences of decisions made now, and yet most pregnancy and birthing decisions are made without investigation into safety, efficacy or rationale. Women do what everyone else does under the assumption that our routine birth practices center around safety and that there is a sound rationale, but that is far from true.

PART THREE-INTERNALIZATION

The realization that birth can be different, followed by why and how of what makes it so *in general* must be followed by reflection of what that means to the individual. What is appropriate for you, specifically? How do you know? What are you doing (or not doing) to create the birth you want? What are your limitations? What limitations have you placed on yourself?

PART FOUR-EXTERNALIZATION

The first three parts are all mental and emotional in nature. By the time the reader finishes Part Three, a paradigm shift should have taken place and now action is required in order to transform the personal experience of birth. To change the outcome, the reader must change her behavior. For some, this may simply mean improving the diet. Others will have come to the realization that in order to increase the likelihood that they will get the birth they know is possible, they will have to make the difficult move to seek out a different provider who holds the same vision of birth that they do.

PART FIVE-REALIZATION

In the best of all possible worlds, everything comes together in the realization of your own best birth! You've done the inner work and you've set up the supportive conditions for your birth ideal to manifest. The combination of mother's intuition, woman's wisdom, nature's design and appropriately applied technology come together in the best way possible.

There are many mothers who thought they prepared a firm foundation only to have it crumble in the end. Why? What pitfalls might prevent the birth that Nature intended? When things don't go the way we planned, when might we acknowledge that we did the best with what we had? When do we learn from the experience and declare, "Never again!" or come to terms with a situation that simply was not in anyone's control? How do we heal in either instance? And regardless of what happens in our own births, do we have a responsibility to the mothers that come after us? Will we joyfully share our stories of painless or orgasmic birth? Should we share stories of how we failed to ask questions we didn't know we should ask, so that other mothers will know they need to ask?

It is my sincere hope that for those mothers that seek a more empowering birth for themselves and a gentler welcome for their babies, this book will be the blueprint that allows them to create it, step-by-step.

18

Introduction

Childbirth books are plentiful. Sadly many books on gentle birth are dismissed, while others that exist only to create compliant patients are given out at doctor's visits and are read with no application of critical thinking skills. The most amazing rationalizations are given as to why books that directly contradict scientific evidence are chosen over those that are supported by evidence. We will explore how and why some women dismiss books that hold the key to better birth.

Ultimately, though some women want gentle birth, many do not believe it's really possible. In general, people avoid concepts that challenge core beliefs. Therefore, a woman who is fearful of birth might dismiss experts in natural childbirth, labeling them as 'naturalists' or 'alarmists,' which makes them easy to write off. Some women insist that to suggest birth can be joyful or comfortable is to be deceitful; to suggest our current system has flaws is seen as nearly heretical. Ignoring accurate information doesn't make it less accurate; disparaging those willing to share facts doesn't change the facts either. This is, basically 'shooting the messenger.'

This book puts forth some very concrete and positive steps to creating the best birth possible for the reader. In order to implement these steps, the rationale for them needs to be established. This means it's imperative to first acknowledge, and then define, the problems that currently exist so that the solutions make sense. I have struggled with how to do this in the most positive way. What I have decided to do is to simply rely on the results; scientific evidence. I will speak to the success or failure of what is currently considered the 'norm' and let the individual decide what makes sense.

To a reader who has been tempted to disregard works that suggest there is an easier way to approach pregnancy, birth and early parenting than what is typical, I would ask, 'Why?' What would be the ulterior motive behind the 'breast is best' or 'there are benefits to natural birth' message? I have actually read articles, full of animosity, which declare that breastfeeding advocates are 'nipple-Nazis' with an agenda. Where does such vehement emotion come from that such violent language would be used? What might be the ulterior motive behind either of these messages, exactly? Really, I ask the reader to consider this. I implore the readers of this book to consider that maybe, just maybe, there is truth in these messages. Act 'as if' there might be legitimacy to the idea that nature has a plan for survival, and that any such plan would have to make a mother's life easier the vast majority of the time if the species were to proliferate. If, after you are finished with the book and actually done the work, you still don't believe that birth can be wonderful, that's fine. I have no problem in agreeing to disagree. It's your birth to do your way. However, I would speculate that you've picked up this book to help you create a better birth. That goal is attainable if you go into this with a willing heart.

For years childbirth options eroded at an appalling pace, leading to an astronomical rise in the rate of surgical birth. By 2009 34% of women would be surgically delivered. (Reinberg, 2011) Despite this, outcomes, meaning the number of mothers and babies that die, do not improve beyond a 5%-10% cesarean rate. (Childbirth Connection, 2011) Since the first edition of *Mother's Intention*, both maternal and infant mortality statistics have worsened. In 2003, data from the August 2002 March of Dimes Perinatal Data Center showed 27 countries had fewer babies dying than the US. That was worse than when I began teaching childbirth education classes in 1990. In 2011 March of Dimes included a world ranking only for maternal mortality (death). There are currently 33 countries with better maternal outcomes, according to this source, but the Safe Motherhood Quilt Project, using World Health Organization (WHO) statistics, states at least 40 countries have better maternal outcomes. Neither statistic is reassuring.

Regarding infant mortality, a rate of 6.9 deaths per 1,000 live births was included in *March of Dimes Foundation Data Book for Policy Makers*. (March of Dimes, 2009) The CIA World Factbook ranks the

U.S., indicating that now, 45 countries have fewer babies die than the U.S. Please take a moment to think about that. We use more routine technology now than 8 years ago, and we still fell in world ranking from 28th to 46th.

Mothers have given away their births. If you want to reclaim joyous birth, I want to put the control back in your hands.

Is it surprising to consider that most women currently don't have control over their births? As you read that sentence, were you tempted to reject the very idea? Was your first reaction to rationalize that maybe other women don't have options, but you certainly do? If so, then you need this book. Or, did you nod your head in agreement that certainly, you have no choice but to do whatever your care-provider tells you, even if it's contrary to common sense? Then you need this book more. Or did you wonder why any woman would *want* control over the most important experience in her life? After all, isn't that the doctor's job? You need this book most of all.

Why do I passionately advocate for gentle birth? Believe me, I ask myself that question on a regular basis! My childbearing days are gone. I had my own best birth. Why have I put the time and energy into your babies by writing, lecturing, and teaching? There's always a pay-off. What's mine? I don't own a breast-milk bank. There's no way for me to hold stock in endorphins or prolactin, just a couple of the body's natural 'feel good' hormones that are part of the 'hormonal blueprint of birth' Dr. Sarah Buckley speaks of in her work. The fact that my husband calls this my 'expensive hobby' may indicate what the financial reward has been. I don't get a fiscal incentive for 'converting' someone to a midwife-attended birth, nor am I rewarded with expensive gifts for support of holistic doctors (though, hey, I'm open to the possibility). I am very proud of the parenting decisions my husband and I have made, confident that they were right for us and most of all, our grown daughter. Of course, that particular confidence comes with our current perspective wherein we are the proud parents of a beautiful, productive, intelligent and witty adult daughter. I also have to say that it is our belief that all of those wonderful attributes that belong to our daughter are hers alone. We were simply blessed with the opportunity to support and nourish her authentic self...or not.

Anyway, the point is, I've done my thing. I'm not looking for support or company in any sort of self-aggrandizing, exclusive group. I don't even think the way I mothered my child is right for everyone. Most of our parenting decisions were based on some solid science, but I also know that every situation calls for individualized problem solving.

I will admit to living vicariously through mothers who glowingly rave about the birth they originally thought impossible. I experience again the wonderment of my own birth. I also like being around these gently born children who exhibit impulse control, compassion and empathy, just as scientists researching undisturbed brain development suggested they would. I feel good knowing these kids will impact my world, and the world my child inherits, in a positive way.

Every time I've been ready to just hang up my teaching hat and focus on a more mundane (and less challenging) day job, someone has told me I helped them change their life. Someone told me the day I sat down to write the original introduction to *Mother's Intention*. When I know that someone's birth was an act of empowerment that helped a family bond into a beautiful thing, because of something I shared, it keeps me going.

My objective is to reduce irrational fear so that women can have the best birth they can have. A fear that is disproportionate to the actual risk is irrational. Fear of birth is completely out of proportion, as you will see if you do the journal exercises in this book, agreeing to keep an open mind about the facts you will read.

The facts may seem irreconcilable with our cultural expectations regarding birth. However, by the end of the book you should be seeing the possibilities available to you in a whole new light.

22

Entire chapters are devoted to issues of fear, guilt and motivation behind many controversies within the 'birthing community.' I ask that the reader take a few days to mull over what they've read in each chapter and to do the work. The material is nothing new, but it may be new to you. It asks, for your own health and well-being and that of your baby, that you entertain thoughts you may never have considered. Some thoughts are contrary to popular belief. I will ask you to look deeply into beliefs you may currently hold as self-evident truths.

You can take control of what is controllable in birth, which is a great deal. This is how guilt is avoided…by being secure in the knowledge that you've made decisions based on all of the information available and with the best of intent. If you want a great birth, do what those have great births do...instead of what everyone else does.

During pregnancy and in the early years of parenting, if you don't become knowledgeable it could affect your life in a big way. When you are knowledgeable, no one can take advantage of you. It's much easier to do the work ahead of time. By reading this book you won't be one of the increasing numbers of women asking, "Why didn't anyone tell me?" I'm telling you, right now.

The question is, are you ready to listen?

PART ONE

Inspiration

ARE YOUR BELIEFS ABOUT BIRTH CONSTRUCTED OF PERCEPTUAL REALITY OR FACTUAL REALITY? HOW DO YOU KNOW THE DIFFERENCE? HOW DOES WHAT YOU BELIEVE ABOUT BIRTH AFFECT YOUR BIRTH? WHAT CAN YOU DO TO BRING YOUR BELIEFS IN LINE WITH SCIENCE SO THAT YOU MIGHT BE INSPIRED TO REACH HIGHER? IS IT POSSIBLE TO ENJOY GIVING BIRTH?

CHAPTER 1

Clearing the Way

We all have a common objective...healthy, happy mother-babies. Used to its highest good, this book can save you time, effort, money, embarrassment, injury and maybe even a life.

Clear communication is essential if the reader is to maximally benefit from this work, so let's take a moment to clarify some terminology that's often tossed about quite casually.

Because it is human nature to assume others are like ourselves, we talk about birth with the assumption that we are all talking about the same experience. Differing birth philosophies mean we may not be, making for emotionally charged exchanges if we don't first take this step.

Even though the majority of birth professionals go out of their way to use neutral language, inevitably miscommunication develops around such personal issues if terminology is not defined. It's human nature to become defensive if a dearly held belief is being challenged. Nowhere are our beliefs held as deeply as those relating to childbirth and childrearing.

Certain terms are inappropriately applied to natural birth advocates on a regular basis. This misuse of language has even spawned new, judgmental terminology, which is interesting, because they stem from the charge that natural birth advocates are 'judgmental.'

Women on natural childbirth (or breastfeeding, or attachment parenting) internet message boards are often accused of being judgmental, so as we examine the definitions of certain words and the misapplication of those words, it might be prudent to begin with the word *'judgmental.'*

The actual meaning of 'judgmental' includes the formation of an authoritative opinion based on comparison of facts. The way it is commonly used, however, often shows a complete lack of discernment on the person leveling the charge, as when the charge is leveled against advocates of natural childbirth, breastfeeding and attachment parenting as mentioned above. Considering there is a great deal of scientific evidence to support the practices mentioned, that seems like an odd charge to level, but it's done all the time.

So, let's roll with the inappropriate use, since it's so pervasive. Even then, more often than not, I see women sharing helpful, evidence-based information that they have personally benefited from, only to be called 'judgmental' for sharing...even when it was shared in the most loving tone, with all sorts of caveats regarding the acknowledgment of special circumstances, etc. Are there self-righteous people out there? Absolutely. Yet, more often than not, the angry respondent is actually feeling defensive and lashing out. We'll explore more about those feelings after we've got consensus on language.

Next, let's look at the idea that the best information is 'balanced' information. If something is balanced, it makes two parts exactly equal so that someone can make a judgment (in the actual meaning of the term) or a decision. It means that the information provided counter-balances or equalizes, bringing something into harmony or proportion. Common usage regarding childbirth and parenting information might be: "I chose the hospital class because they provide balanced information."

Thus, truly balanced childbirth information would include all birth options *or* would provide information that is missing from the commonly available information in order to provide real balance. I've taught hospital childbirth classes, and I can tell you I was *not allowed* to give balanced information at one institution. I was at another. If a childbirth class talks about the benefits of epidurals but minimizes the risks, that's not balance. If a woman is required to sign a document outlining the risks of a vaginal birth after cesarean

(VBAC), but not one regarding the risks of repeat surgery, she is not being given balanced information. This book provides balance in that it exposes the reader to a number options and ideas that are given short shrift in our current system, not that it provides 'both sides' of any issue of the childbearing year. The prevailing childbearing information is already so one-sided that most people don't even question it. Here, we question it, but we do so by simply asking what evidence supports the status quo.

To some, this may seem to present a biased perspective. I would assert exactly the opposite. Although I certainly recognize that I have a bias, after more than 20 years of research, I have what I feel is sufficient knowledge on which to base my prejudices.

People dismiss some of the best, most unbiased and balanced childbirth books with comments like, "I didn't find that book useful because it was so biased" which often means, "This book does not fit with what I already believe" even if all options are equally examined by the author.

As examples, the following books are very fact-based: *Gentle Birth Choices*, by Barbara Harper (which gives equal time to all options), and *The Thinking Woman's Guide to Better Birth* or *Obstetric Myths versus Research Realities*, both by Henci Goer (both weigh current practice against the scientific literature).

Have you ever heard of these books? Have you read them? Why or why not? Do the books you are reading fairly represent all options? If the picture you get of safe birth is only that which is currently culturally acceptable in the United States, they are not.

What if all available options are not equal? What if a parent will be making decisions that will affect both herself and her baby with both short and long term consequences. Is it fair to distort reality so that the information she has to choose from seems 'equal,' even though it really isn't? Why would a parent want information that appears balanced, but isn't factual?

The most popular books maintain the status quo and very often are not supported by evidence...do not give "equal force or influence to" proven safe options such as home-birth or freestanding birth centers. By "informing" women that they can *expect* substandard care, women *accept* substandard care.

When it comes to childbirth classes, there are many options. If asked why they chose a childbirth class at the hospital instead of an independent class, some parents maintain it's more "balanced."

Consider this:

In a hospital class the childbirth educator (CBE) is an employee of the hospital. She may only teach pre-approved material. She may not be able to fully answer questions posed by parents if the response contradicts the protocols of the hospital, or even one doctor, no matter if she can provide scientific evidence for her answer and the doctor cannot. (This actually happened to me more often than you may want to believe while I was teaching in-hospital.) An instructor in an institution cannot give unbiased, balanced information that includes any providers other than those who sign her checks. Think about it from the hospital's point of view. Would you hire someone who would provide information that might help parents take their dollars elsewhere? As a doctor, would you send your patients to a class where they might learn there are other caregivers who practice under safer guidelines?

Classes in the hospital are actually more affordable because of the bias under which they operate. Formula, drug and diaper companies often subsidize these classes. Look at the teaching materials you receive. In small print, on the back, you will often find a pharmaceutical company, disposable diaper or baby food logo. The content of the class can be determined in large part by how involved other parties are. The 'free' gifts are rarely 'free.'

An independent instructor is not subsidized. Her passion for birth usually (though certainly not always) happened one of two ways—

either she had such a horrible birth experience she went on a mission to discover what went wrong and now wants to spare you her anguish, or she had such a wonderful birth experience she wants to share the steps to better birth she used. I'm the latter, in case you wondered.

With an independent instructor, you sign her paycheck. She can fully and honestly answer any question you ask. She works as a CBE because she wants to make a difference, not because she's grudgingly been assigned the task on top of her long OB nursing shift.

In fact, she may not even be a nurse, which is to your advantage. Nursing is a highly skilled profession requiring an enormous amount of knowledge from pediatrics to geriatrics; surgical to pharmaceutical. Normal labor and birth are a very small part of what they learn in their extensive training, and an even smaller part of their experience if the only births they ever witness are medically managed. Again, through personal experience I can tell you there are nurses who have worked for *years* before ever witnessing a truly natural birth.

An independent CBE is an autonomous practitioner who only studies pregnancy, birth and (sometimes) early parenting. Because her specialty is quite narrow, she knows more about what you need to know. Her education likely included study of all birth options, as does her continuing education.

An independent instructor has compared and contrasted every option available to pregnant mothers. Having done so, her classes are most likely 'natural childbirth' classes.

Parents often think that's what their hospital class is. If it's called a 'prepared childbirth' class or an 'expectant parent' class, it's not. Again, I've taught both. I know.

Even a class billed 'natural childbirth' may not be what it seems. There is confusion over what 'natural childbirth' means, which is why I include it here in the list of terms to clarify. For some, a 'natural birth' is a birth as nature intended, simple, unaltered by man, devoid of drugs and surgery. For others, a natural birth is any vaginal birth and the suggestion that the interventions are not natural is (while undeniably true) somehow insulting.

Why? Because, it is explained, someone who views nature birth so narrowly is not being objective. Cultural and personal ideas about what constitutes 'natural' may differ, but the very definition of the word simply is what is. There is no judgment implied in declaring something as nature designed it. To point that out is not to distort fact insert personal feeling or prejudice. Could a vaginal birth with natural (produced by nature) interventions such as nipple stimulation, positional changes or relaxation techniques be considered 'natural?' I would consider it so.

"I COULDN'T FIGURE OUT WHY WOMEN WERE RUSHING OUT TO LEARN WHAT TO EXPECT INSTEAD OF LEARNING TO EXPECT BETTER."
KIM WILDNER

Is pitocin made by nature? No. Does it affect the natural process of birth? Yes. Are drugs such as Stadol, Nubain or Demerol made in nature? No. Do they affect the natural process? Yes. Are epidural drugs made by nature? No. Do they affect normal labor progression? Yes.

It would stand to reason then, that while a vaginal birth is possible with such alterations of the birth process, deeming all vaginal births natural is a stretch.

Please note that restoring the term 'natural childbirth' to its actual meaning does not 'take' anything away from any woman who wishes to reframe her own experience. It simply brings the term back into compliance with the definition of 'natural' for the sake of clear communication. Perception is reality. Some prefer to call surgical births 'natural.'

I am choosing to use natural in the literal sense.

Also, note that in doing so, no judgment has been implied. Distinction of natural birth, vaginal birth and surgical birth simply means they are dissimilar. There is no doubt that they are different experiences. Not better or worse, just different.

Thus, just because someone doesn't agree with the facts does not mean they are not being presented with objective information. It just means they disagree with the facts, which is their prerogative.

We can't have a discussion about birth if we are not on the same page, so to speak.

Do some of the words we've looked at, misused or not, accurately describe natural birth and parenting advocates? Sadly, yes. I would contend no more so than they describe anyone else, however; perhaps less so from my own personal experience. More often, though, I see people ascribing motivations and judgment where none is intended.

What about the information about to be presented in this book? It is biased? Judgmental? Objective? How are these words used in heated debate and whom does it harm?

Even having taken great pains to use neutral language and explicitly state that different only means different, experience dictates that there will be a few people who will read 'better/worse, good/bad, always/never' where it does not exist. If your initial reaction is to do so, please take a moment to consider why. We come to our current thinking due to past experiences and knowledge. Why people chose to take offense where none is intended is a complex issue, but I won't deny that for some reason mothers seem more prone to offense. I wish that were not the case.

Birth does not place us in competition with other women. We do that to ourselves. Birth is the most singular experience with our true self that we can have. In the following example, see how removal of the personal element by using a different experience shifts perception, thus reality.

How about if we take it out of the medical realm? Since birth is usually not a medical event or illness, it may be more appropriate to use an example of marathon participants, where the objective is to test one's endurance, finishing the race, but not necessarily first. Pride comes from the accomplishment of working hard to achieve a goal. There are no losers.

One person trained hard all year, eating well and exercising daily.
One person does the same, with the addition that he requires insulin to treat a diabetic condition, or any medication for any medical condition.
One person does the same, aided by a prosthesis replacing a lost limb.
One person does the same from a wheel chair due to paraplegia.
One sort of prepares, but decides part way through the race to catch a ride to the finish line.

All the same experience? No. There is no shame in finishing a race assisted by modern medicine when necessary. Indeed, those people must overcome obstacles others never even face. Should the person who *could not have* functioned without assistance of wheels be viewed the same as someone who choses them? How fair is it to the person who worked so hard to be put in the same category as someone who makes the decision not to? If the only goal is to cross the finish line, who is to judge how one gets there? The only opinion that matters is the participant's. Who is to determine how a participant should feel? Who decides who will be allowed to say they did it 'on their own?' Must we all agree on a definition of 'success', or is reality wholly the participant's perception?

How did it come to be that the definition of 'natural childbirth' came to include the very antithesis of 'natural?'

34

Intentionally. By manipulating language, we manipulate experience. 'Natural' should mean 'that which comes naturally.' By calling the obstetrically managed experience 'normal' despite the many non-medially indicated, inappropriately applied interventions used, those interventions then come to be seen as 'natural' because most people equate 'natural' with 'normal.' This is the progression of how flat-on-the-back births with IVs, drugs, inductions and episiotomies came to be accepted as 'normal.' Birth has been re-conceptualized, re-labeled and re-marketed. It's up to mothers to reclaim natural birth.

In order to do that, mothers have to stop arguing over what is 'natural.' I propose the following commonsense definitions:

Natural birth: Birth not made or altered by man; being such by nature.
Vaginal birth: Birth wherein the baby passes though the birth passage, regardless of interventions used. A natural birth is a vaginal birth, but a vaginal birth may not be a natural birth.
Surgical birth: Birth wherein the baby is surgically removed from the mother's uterus.

"RE-EXAMINE ALL THAT YOU HAVE BEEN TOLD... DISMISS THAT WHICH INSULTS YOUR SOUL."
WALT WHITMAN

All terms use the word 'birth'; no term is inflammatory or derogatory; all are accurate and honest.

Honesty is frequently (and erroneously) called 'judgmental' when the subject is birth or parenting. There are two important things to consider before rejecting pregnancy, birthing and parenting information.

One must first ask, "Was the intent of the person sharing said information malicious or benevolent?" then "Did the language actually contain judgment words, or did I hear judgment words?" and finally "If no judgment was intended or implied, why did I hear it? Is there self-judgment, or am I projecting judgment?"

Actual 'judgmental attitudes', the negative meaning usually ascribed to the term, are easy to spot and quite different from simple honesty when the two are compared and contrasted. I don't know a childbirth professional who would ever make judgmental comments to any mother like those found in the second group that follows, though I know many who have been accused of saying those things when what actually they said was something similar to the neutral comments first presented. I won't claim that no one, professional or not, ever passes judgment in a negative way, only that the accusation is most often unfounded.

Judgmental statements use judgmental words and blanket statements...bad, good, crazy, idiot, horrible, selfish, always, never. Shoot, just typing them made me feel bad. Please be aware that I do not hold the opinions given as 'judgmental!' I do not know anyone who does. I have heard them mistaken for the honest statements, which is why I chose to use them as examples.

Honest phrases:

There is no medical reason for routine circumcision.
There is no artificial mother's milk substitute that is as good for babies as mother's milk.
Epidurals have short and long-term negative effects on both mother and baby.
Natural birth means "as nature intended."

Judgmental phrases:

Genital mutilation is abuse.
Women who don't breastfeed are selfish.
Mothers who need epidurals are wimps.
It's idiotic to call an induced or epidural birth "natural."

Who talks to other people that way? I will say I have rarely heard it, but more often than not when someone is accused of being judgmental what was actually said and what the listener heard are two very different things. However, people often hard on themselves and project their own feelings onto another.

Judgments are based on opinion and therefore cannot be substantiated. Anyone who hears them would be offended. Honest statements, on-the-other-hand, are made with neutral language. They contain verifiable truth. Honest statements do not hold judgment, though the judgmental may hold some truth, which is where people may get confused.

Honest statements may be heard as judgmental by someone who is judgmental, but not by everyone. An objective bystander hearing an honest statement might wonder why it would upset anyone.

An objective bystander would be hard to find, though, since we all see the world through the lens of our personal experience. We all form opinions from the time we begin absorbing our environment. Some of our opinions we have formulated on our own through experience, some we have inherited. This colors incoming messages. If we hear malice or judgment where it does not exist, it is the lens we currently use that distorts what we allow into our reality construct.

What if there is malice intended? What if a truly vicious person makes a comment with the sole intent of making another person feel bad for no reason?

It's still all about the malicious person holding the judgment, whose reality is created by the lens that distorts their perception. Their judgment has nothing to do with anyone but them. Even if the judgment is directed at me, I know the person holding the judgment feels that way about everyone, all the time. If I don't take it personally, it doesn't have to hurt me. I can choose to ignore it, realizing it has nothing to do with me. Only you can decide if you will choose to let it mean anything to you.

Do you care what a stranger thinks about your birth? Do you care what anyone thinks about your choices? Why? How liberating it is to be able to step back and not take someone else's perception of reality personally. It takes an awful lot of energy to be offended by comments with no offense behind them, and isn't it also a little arrogant to think that the choices we make regarding birth are of concern to anyone but ourselves? By making assumptions and taking things personally, we only hurt ourselves.

Every person has a lens. Every opinion is biased, including the ones you hold. The question is, what created the perception leading to a particular bias? Does the bias benefit you or not? Is the bias warranted? Does your own bias prevent access of information that might benefit you? Is your bias based on fact?

If someone were to pass judgment on you for something you didn't do or something you felt confident about, do you think you'd feel defensive, guilty or hurt? Not likely. You would simply shrug off the comment or the person making it. For example, if someone were to brand you as 'elitist' or insisted you were wasting your time and/or money going to college, but you know you need the degree to get the job you want, would you feel guilty and drop out? Not likely, because that person has little understanding of what is necessary for you.

One last human tendency that gets in the way of clear communication is making assumptions, especially from a 'right' or 'wrong', 'good' or 'bad' mind-set. This has created an enormous chasm between those trying to help women create better births and the women themselves.

Is 'better' a judgment word? Only if it is applied in the context of 'my birth was better than your birth.' We need to stop this 'competition' between mothers!

Current birth management is leaving mothers feeling that they can't cope, with war stories instead of joyful birth stories. Current birth and parenting advice, in the noble attempt to not offend anyone, gives advice that helps no one. We can do better. That is how I use the term.

In any case, assuming one personal choice makes another one wrong distorts communication about the choices themselves.

It is often assumed by some that if a mother has a home birth she hates doctors and hospitals.

Truth: The vast majority of home birth mothers recognize that hospitals and doctors are necessary in special circumstances. If they were sick or injured in pregnancy, they would not hesitate to gratefully utilize technology.

It is often assumed that because natural birth advocates want parents to have truthful information about labor drugs they are against compassionate use of, or medically indicated pharmaceuticals.

Truth: Not so...only unnecessary or inappropriate used, without full disclosure of risk.

Mothers face judgment for how they birth and parent every day. Not all choose to take offense. No one can make someone feel something they do not choose to feel. A woman who is confident that she has made her own best choices for herself and her family, based on the best information that could be found at the time, isn't the least bit interested in anyone else's opinion. Why would she be concerned if anyone agrees with her or care about how anyone else's feelings about what she does? She could attempt to explain her decisions, but people making assumptions and judgments don't actually want to hear about solid decision making strategies if it conflicts with what they already believe to be true. They don't even hear, much less listen or consider.

As you work through this book and perhaps start making decisions that may be different from what our society considers the norm, you may hear comments with a lot of anger and hurt behind them, seemingly directed at you. Comments like, "Well I did [such and such] and my kids are just fine!" when you never implied that they weren't. You may never even had a thought in your head that the other person could have or should have done anything differently, but they are seeing your actions though their own lens and making assumptions. It doesn't have anything to do with your choices or why you made them.

In fact, if you tried to explain why you made a particular decision, they probably won't even hear you because they aren't upset about you and your decision...they have issues with their own decisions. They are stuck in an either/or mind-set.

'IF FIFTY MILLION PEOPLE SAY A FOOLISH THING, IT IS STILL A FOOLISH THING."
ANATOLE FRANCE

If you think your decision is right, the assumption is you think their decision was wrong. It's best to just let it go. We are only responsible for our own heath and well-being.

It is true that those of use who have been trying to improve the safety and experience of birth for decades get frustrated when we hear story-after-potentially-preventable-tragic-story. We want so much better for women and babies, not because we're judgmental or think that every birth can (or should) be the same, but because we've seen so much sorrow that didn't have to happen!

If you were psychic and could foretell a train wreck about to happen, would you be frustrated that a person ignored your warning and was hurt?

If your adult self could go back and tell your child self what you know now so that her life could be better, would you? Would you be aggravated if she didn't listen?

Natural birth supporters aren't trying to scare you by telling you what you don't want to hear; we are trying to help you! What you don't know can hurt you! If you don't know your options, you don't

40

have any. If you make decisions that net the expected, with all the unhappiness mothers now complain of, we are sad that you have to endure that...not judgmental. Closing one's eyes to the truth does not make it cease to exist...it only makes one powerless to deal with the reality.

Which brings us to 'objective.' Natural birth advocates are often passionate about natural birth. Passion does not preclude objectivity. If a person's personal opinion is based on emotion alone, then obviously they are not objective. However, if their passion arises from facts 'existing outside and independent of the mind' and there is no distortion of the facts 'by personal feelings or prejudice', then the information is quite objective. How does one know the difference? Test the validity of the assertion. In this work, I have provided the resources to do just that in the notes. Yes, I'm passionate. I'm also objective. I've even been known to change my mind in the face of evidence!

So, who am I, and why would what I have to say matter?

I am you. I am a daughter, a wife, a mother. I grew up in the Midwest in the typical American family with 2.2 children. I was influenced by the same cultural ideas about pregnancy and birth that most people have.

The 'point two' child came into my family when I was 12 years old. As a strong willed child prone to testing the data, I questioned everything my mother went through. I wanted to know 'why' to everything. I found it strangely disconcerting that there were no logical answers to my questions. Even the answers that were supposed to be logical didn't compute.

Why would a woman need to be cut (an episiotomy) to get a baby out? If nature were so incompetent as to make the birth passage inadequate to birth a baby, why weren't all mammals walking around with damaged vaginas? As it seemed to me, only human mothers were…due to the episiotomy! There were dozens of other illogical (to me) rituals in becoming a mother. Often the only 'reason' for them was because "That's what they do." (Ah! The ubiquitous 'they!')

My husband and I were faced with infertility when we decided to start our family. It took us 5 years to get pregnant the first time. That pregnancy ended in miscarriage. Our only child, a daughter, was conceived a year later. In attempting to better understand everything I could about infertility and reproduction, I did a lot of research, which led to information about midwifery.

I began to learn that my original instincts about birth were right. Not only was there no good reason behind much of the technology routine in modern birth, but much of it was actually proven harmful. I began a path toward midwifery, certain that with all of the information available…information that eventually enabled me to have a wonderful, safe birth without being cut, poked or drugged once we finally conceived…women would soon be looking for ways to have empowering births like mine.

In the 80's and 90's a plethora of unproven technologies continued to be unleashed on women with no improvement in outcomes, many with serious questions of not only efficacy but safety. Women became more fearful than ever. The harder those of us in the know tried to impart vital knowledge, the faster women ran toward the burning barn. I couldn't figure out why women were rushing out to learn what to expect instead of learning to expect better. It took me years to figure out the reason. It had nothing to do with facts and everything to do with belief.

I set aside my midwifery aspirations to concentrate on what had, at first, been a steppingstone to midwifery…education. I focused my attention on writing and teaching. Still, the ones who 'got it' were few-and-far-between. I felt like I was spinning my wheels. Why couldn't I get through to these intelligent parents?

I couldn't get around their fear.

Whether consciously acknowledged or unconscious in nature, until the fear is dealt with, the belief holds firm. I educated myself on how to release false assumptions and applied critical thinking skills to our common cultural beliefs about birth. *Mother's Intention* sprang to life.

If used in pregnancy, birth and early parenthood, success—and by results this means the safest birth possible for you and the easiest transition into parenthood—is inevitable.

You will find that this material is based on evidence-based care...and that what you think you know just isn't so when it comes to maternity care in the US. I feel a duty to use my life to educate women on evidence-based care, which they believe is what they are getting. Women in America today are basing life-altering decisions on belief that they think is fact. Each subsequent decision is affected by that very first belief. Everything I share will be substantiated so that the reader can research the data. Not only do I encourage it, I expect it.

Sometimes wisdom comes from odd sources...I live by this little gem I found on a tube of lip balm years ago and later discovered to be a Walt Whitman quote: "Re-examine all that you have been told... dismiss that which insults your soul."

Being Honest about Motherhood

In September of 2002, daytime talk featured shows on the difficulties mothers face today, from dealing with postpartum depression and the loss of 'self' to not wanting to be mothers at all. It was agreed that mothers are in crisis. They are having trouble coping. Many are disillusioned that no one told them how hard this job was.

- 32-34 % OF BIRTHS ARE SURGICAL, UP FROM 25% IN 2003.
- IN A HARRIS POLL CONDUCTED BY THE MATERNITY CENTER ASSOCIATION, THERE WERE NO NATURAL BIRTHS IN THE STUDY, DESPITE THE FACT THAT 45% SAID THEY AGREED WITH THE STATEMENT THAT "GIVING BIRTH IS A NATURAL PROCESS THAT SHOULD NOT BE INTERFERED WITH UNLESS MEDICALLY NECESSARY."
- WOMEN ARE SO AFRAID OF BIRTH THEY ARE FUELING THESE SELF-DESTRUCTIVE TRENDS.
- WOMEN ARE FORMING SUPPORT GROUPS TO 'GET THROUGH' THE WEEKS OR MONTHS IT IS TAKING THEM TO LOVE THEIR BABIES, DECLARING THAT BONDING IS A MYTH BECAUSE THEY DIDN'T EXPERIENCE IT.
- WOMEN ARE SAYING THEIR BREASTS ARE BLEEDING DUE TO NORMAL USAGE IN THE PHYSIOLOGICAL FUNCTION FOR WHICH THEY WERE DESIGNED, YET ALL OTHER MAMMALS USE THEM WITHOUT INCIDENT.

Some are angry at the discovery that motherhood is not a task that fits neatly between day jobs and isn't even a simple day job itself.

They feel unable to deal with the problems and challenges with which they are faced, assuming they are somehow deficient. They wonder how other mothers do it, or they insist the mothers who say they love mothering and find it pretty easy are lying. Some may be faced with challenges they didn't sign up for. Even more have created problems where none would have existed but for the choices they made, yet our 'feel good' society is loathe to point that out for fear of seeming to 'mother bash.' How can anyone learn from their mistakes if everyone is too afraid point out that the mistakes exist?! The emperor is naked, people!

If you are one of the mothers feeling overwhelmed, you may feel it's unfair that your life seems out of control. Maybe it is. I don't want to minimize the magnitude of the job. It is enormous. It's the best job in the world, but that doesn't mean you'll love doing it 24/7. The fact remains that it is what it is and you need to find a way to manage it. You need to know what you are culpable for so that next time around you don't make the same mistakes. Most women will only get a couple of cracks at this motherhood thing.

This book won't tell you what to expect. What you can expect will change based on your own actions and the set of circumstances presented to you. Without action behind intent, there is no grow, no change. You get what you put into it, for better or for worse.

An open mind is essential for creating the birth you want. Letting go of resistance is imperative. Believe me when I say that there will be long held ideas that will be challenged. Give the new ideas a fair chance. Test their accuracy and validity.

For most parents-to-be, someone else is controlling your outcome. Parents are just rolling along with no plan, leaving the most important work with which they'll ever be entrusted to chance. These parents will live with the consequences of their choices for a lifetime, yet decisions are made without true informed consent or worse, under duress as their fear and love for their baby is played upon.

Are you holding yourself, or those making life-and-death decisions for you, to the highest standards? Does every decision ask, "What is in the best interest of the child?" whenever and wherever possible? Or, are you doing what 'everyone else' does just because everyone else does?

How did we get here?

We didn't arrive by accident at this place where common sense is uncommon in obstetrical care. The progression is easy to dissect and examine.

Human behavior in obstetricians is the same as in the rest of us. Some of the traits we will explore in ourselves (and in these human beings who have bore the weight of our perceptions) are not pleasant to face.

It is necessary though, because nowhere else are they more damaging than in our experience as parents. For as a parent, you are not only accountable for your own life, but the life you have created, and, by extension, all the lives that life touches. Talk about a ripple effect!

Very pulled together people, people who excel in every other area of their lives, still will not ask themselves the questions that beg to be asked regarding parenthood. Mothers are drowning in guilt already, so it's become politically incorrect to talk about accountability. "Of course, it's a choice" we say of so much of parenting, and of course it is. But few are willing to say that some choices create problems that otherwise might not have existed. This is unfair to the mothers who are yet to come, implying that all choices are equal, when they simply are not. It cheats them out of the opportunity to make the better choice. It is a symptom of a destructive human trait...denial.

Parents are not immune to the tendency to make assumptions without testing their integrity or accuracy. Every choice made from an erroneous assumption is then flawed. In pregnancy and birth, the consequences can be fatal. Shutting out additional possibilities because of the 'rightness' of what you believe means you fail to see what is available to you. Thinking that stems from this may seem logical, but the conclusions are wrong. Just because you want something to be true doesn't make it so.

Many obstetricians seem to be stuck in this place. They'd rather be right than be safe. Show them the evidence that 'standard of care' is ineffective or harmful and they will dismiss it, or even manipulate the data to substantiate their position. (Wagner, 2001) Most of the time they aren't questioned.

While *Mother's Intention* was being written, the media carried the news that a study now confirmed that Vaginal Birth After Cesarean (VBAC) was dangerous. They didn't say that it was the same study that ACOG used to support VBAC just a few years earlier, or that there are a multitude of better designed studies that also say VBAC is safer than repeat cesarean. (Goer, 2002) It didn't take long…not even weeks…for this recommendation to become 'we need to support elective cesarean." I warned then, "Watch the numbers of surgical births…they are about to skyrocket." Indeed, as predicted, this is exactly what happened. The rate went from about 24% in 2003 to 32-34% in 2011.) This is not a good thing. I hope that by the end of this book you will understand why.

The human tendency to assume can color how the above information and that which follows is interpreted.

Therefore, it needs to be clear from the outset that information provided on evidenced-based care and the dangers of 'obstetrical management,' is critical of a broken system that is statistically, scientifically and experientially not working, not a condemnation of the doctors, midwives, nurses or childbirth educators within that system. No comment is being made on any particular institutions within that system. There are shining stars trying to fix what's broken from the inside, and their work is difficult. If you are one of the fortunate that cannot reconcile your experience with what you are reading, you have probably found one of them. Nominate the institutions in which they work for Mother-Friendly Childbirth Initiative designation through CIMS, the Coalition for Improving Maternity Services.

"NEVER DOUBT THAT A SMALL GROUP OF THOUGHTFUL PEOPLE COULD CHANGE THE WORLD. INDEED, IT'S THE ONLY THING THAT EVER HAS." MARGARET MEAD

Unfortunately, these special people are all too rare. Results don't lie.

Again, unfortunately, this book will benefit those that think they are in the ideal situation, but may not be.

Far too many women who loved their doctors because they were 'nice,' who were assured nothing that wasn't medically necessary would be done, have ended up with the same unacceptable results so many women face everyday. Lulled by a caregiver's reassurance that "...of course pregnancy and birth are a natural process, but..." throughout pregnancy, they are blindsided in the last 6 weeks with one of those 'buts.' There are a multitude of reasons, it seems, to 'get that baby out of there'; baby is too small, too big, too early, too late, too much amniotic fluid, too little fluid. These are all very real concerns...in an extraordinarily small percentage of pregnancies. Yet, an alarmingly high number of women are 'diagnosed' with these conditions. What's a parent to do?

Healthy skepticism is to be encouraged. This does not foster distrust in a healthy relationship with a competent care provider. Asking for evidence beyond 'Because I say so' is reasonable adult behavior when adults must make important decisions. If results back up the words your relationship improves...your trust grows.

For instance, there are a growing number of doctors and nurses within the current non-functioning system that have done their homework and will tell you, if you ask, that an option presented throughout this book, home birth, is a viable option if you are healthy and have a skilled attendant. They will reasonably add that it is not right for every woman, but it is perfectly safe for healthy women with healthy babies.

Still, the 'official' ACOG* opinion, is that home-birth is not safe.

*(American College of Obstetricians and Gynecologists, or as of January 2010, the American Congress of Obstetricians and Gynecologists, which apparently are two different organizations, purposely sharing the same acronym, the same board, the same dues paying members and lobbyists. Confused?)

What is that based on? Why 'studies' of course. However, what most people don't realize is that these 'studies' are virtually identical in their questionable methodology and stand in lonely opposition to every other independent study indicating home birth is as safe as a hospital birth.

In order to get the results they did, one of the earliest studies included abortions, stillbirths, infanticide and unplanned out-of-hospital births...i.e. taxicabs and elevators as well as ..."homicides by unwed mothers who did not want their babies and left them to die of exposure and neglect." (Stewart, 1981)

Not quite a fair representation. Two more recent studies often touted in the media are the Pang (Pang et al, 2002) and Wax (Wax et al, 2010) studies.

Upon the evaluation of the Pang study, it was found that "Method of selection did not distinguish between the planned home births, out-of-hospital births that had no attendant, or births with unknown or unnamed attendants. Premature births occurring between 34 and 37 weeks were incorrectly included in the initial analysis. A higher incidence of congenital heart disease in the home birth population could partially explain the higher neonatal mortality and would reflect a difference in populations." (Vedam, Schummers, & Fulton, 2011)

The Wax study purportedly found a three times greater mortality rate associated with home birth, and the title of the study, "Maternal and newborn outcomes in planned home birth vs planned hospital births: a meta-analysis." might suggest that this would specifically relate to *planned* home birth. However, examination of this study reveals, "The methodology and statistical analysis employed in this systematic review were deeply flawed. This meta-analysis is fraught with calculation errors, with selective and mistaken inclusion/exclusion of studies when analyzing specific outcomes, as well as logical flaws in terms of definitions." (ibid)

So what does this mean? It means that the studies deliberately included information that would create a false impression that home birth was unsafe. It means the numbers were intentionally manipulated. It means that definitions were changed to force conclusions that didn't actually exist.

ACOG has raged an all out war against home birth in the last few years, yet with the exception of the flawed studies they use, all other studies show home birth to have similar, or better, outcomes than hospital birth. For anyone wishing to explore the many studies that support a woman's right to chose where and with whom she might like to birth, James J. Hughes Ph.D. maintains a page, *The Safety of Home Birth,* (Hughes, nd) where the many studies in support of home birth are archived. Ronnie Falco also maintains a page with studies as well as critiques and responses on her Gentle Birth Midwife Archives. (Falco, nd)

Home birth is not the only place where this lack of evidence, or manipulation of evidence, takes place in obstetrics. In August 2011 Obstetrics & Gynecology, the journal of the American College of Obstetricians and Gynecologists, published an article that conceded that only one-third of clinical guidelines for OB/GYN practice are based on "good and consistent scientific evidence." Instead, it was revealed that recommendations for patient care are based on "limited or inconsistent evidence" and on "expert opinion."

An example of one of these unsupported practices is that of routine gestational diabetes testing in the absence symptoms or risk factors. *A Guide to Effective Care in Pregnancy and Childbirth* states, "The available data provides no evidence to support the wide recommendation that all pregnant women should be screened for 'gestational diabetes'..." (pp. 59), and for good reason. *In Understanding Diagnostic Tests in the Childbearing Year* we find that this test is not reproducible 70 out of 100 times! It's not accurate; it's harmful to women (in that it is a 'fasting' blood sugar test, requiring a pregnant woman to go without food for 8-12 hours, and then ingest pure sugar syrup despite the fact that her pregnancy physiology makes her less able to cope with this unnatural overload), yet it is the 'standard of care.'

Another example of nonsensical thinking is the story of a friend who broke her tailbone four days past her estimated due date.

She obviously was in a great deal of pain. At the hospital, she was told all they could give her for the pain was a commonly available pain reliever because anything stronger would be bad for the baby. BUT...if she went into labor, (or if they just would let them induce her), she could have an epidural or Demerol. She responded with, "Excuse me? Why is it not OK to relieve the pain of a pathological condition that is by its very nature painful, but it is OK for a normal, physiological process that can be quite comfortable without drugs?" (More on that later!) If she went into labor in 10-minutes she could have the drug, but not now? How does the difference of 10 minutes make the drug less dangerous? The same rationale makes it not OK for a mother to have narcotics/opiates in her system if she puts it there, but it is OK if the anesthesiologist does? I am not advocating illicit drug use here. I'm simply pointing out officially an estimated 76% (Sakala & Corry, 2008) of our babies are born under the influence of epidurals. Some admit that in their hospitals, the numbers are closer to 90%. (Mothering, 2010) Epidurals are comprised of narcotics and 'caine drugs.

We ignore the nonsensical, the lack of evidence and the disingenuousness in our maternity care system at our own peril. If we do, we make our decisions and base our behavior based on misinformation. If choosing the interventions means choosing the consequences that's a costly mistake to make. If we aren't willing to demand accountability those mistakes are repeated, improving nothing. I hope to help those that expect more of themselves and for their children.

Have you made choices that might be setting you up for an unintended outcome? Is this a second child and you wonder if something you did, or didn't do, created a problem with your first child? Do you wonder if yours was an unnecessary cesarean, or if jaundice was a result of the labor drugs that your baby had to try to process with an immature liver? Angry that no one told you what you didn't dream you would need to ask? You shouldn't have to, but until overall outcomes improve, you do. It's a lot you shouldn't have to shoulder, but you do if you want to be safe. You have no choice at this time in history.

If you are angry about that, I feel the need to say very clearly, find a way to process that anger. I'm not here to judge, but to support and educate. I am here to tell it like it is, which means some people will be facing some painful epiphanies. However, guilt and shame will are pointless. Guilt is meant to be put to use. It's an internal emotion meant to (theoretically) help us modulate our own behavior in a positive way. No one can 'make' you feel guilty if you do not choose to hook into that. If you feel good about your choices, knowing in your heart that your intent was well meaning and you did the best you could there is no purpose in feeling guilty. If you did make the best choice you could with the information you had, and later find out there was another option, you need to ask yourself, "Would I make a different choice next time?" If the answer is 'yes' the feeling of guilt has done what it was meant to do. If the answer is 'no' and rift with excuses or justifications, then it's supposed to nag you.

Either way, what is, is. All you can do is deal with what's before you. You can't change the past. You may be able to compensate or you may need professional help to let it work through your feelings, but holding on to it will eat at your soul.

If you are feeling over-whelmed, that's understandable. We should learn all of this in college, or better yet in high school, so we can enter this most important transition with calm confidence and joy. I'm trying to build that reality for my daughter. I hope you'll help me for the sake of your own daughters as well as yourselves.

Parenthood is the toughest job that you'll ever do. It's also the most rewarding. It begs us to stand alone sometimes, even when we are uncomfortable with it, because our children expect us to be the best we can be. Their lives are in our hands.

Throughout this book, I encourage the reader to examine their thoughts, the origin of their beliefs, and any feelings that may crop up if and when those thoughts and beliefs are challenged. I would suggest a dedicated journal for this work.

Journal Exploration:

Explore the following:

What assumptions or beliefs do you have regarding birth?
Which are you willing to challenge? Is there something you fear about birth and labor?
Are there concerns about new motherhood?
Do you create excuses to justify not making meaningful changes to improve your birth outcome?
If your caregiver is leading you down the path of cascading intervention that leads to an unnecessary cesarean, will you make a stand?
Why or why not?
If you leave the office in tears, unsure, confused, angry or afraid, will you fire that provider and seek out another who supports your vision ob birth?
Why or why not?

There is a high probability that what made this list are things over which you have at least some control, through your thoughts, choices or actions, even if at first your current thinking causes you to resist that idea. Are you afraid of complications in birth? Most preventable complications, and many are preventable, are related to nutrition. Have you learned about how you need to eat to grow a healthy baby? Do you know how sugar impacts your pregnancy health? Have you stopped smoking?

Some complications are seen almost exclusively in obstetrically managed births...have you interviewed midwives, made a birth preference list or do you need to find an OB that shares your birthing philosophy? If you avoid the non-medically indicated intervention, you avoid the complication. Do you know what would constitute a medical indication for specific interventions likely at your place of birth or with your current caregiver?

Do you know what complications are common to certain interventions? Knowing what you have control over allows you to be more accepting of what you don't.

How Important are Parents?

Many of the choices parents make on behalf of their baby with little or no conscious thought, from the childbearing year through the first 3 years, will set the stage for the life the child for as long as they draw breath. From the minute a woman finds out she's pregnant, it is her responsibility to know how her every action and decision...including the food she eats, the prenatal technologies she will utilize, how she births, and what she will feed her child...will impact that child and make her decisions based on the best interest of the child whenever possible.

There has been a five-fold increase in childhood diabetes in the last 10 years that many logically attribute to low breastfeeding rates in the US. (Mirkin, 1999; CBS 2010) Autism has increased by at least 400% in the last 10 to 15 years which some speculate may be due to vaccinations (Null, 2011) and others to mothers who smoke or to inappropriate prenatal and birth technology such as routine ultrasound and immediate clamping/cutting of the umbilical cord.

54

(Beech & Robinson, 1994; Wagner, 1999; Sepkoski, Lester, Osthemimer& Brazelton, 1992) Other autoimmune disorders, like MS, are also on the rise, with suspected origins in infancy or early childhood. Life threatening allergies are such a problem that schools have 'peanut free' zones. Is it coincidence that the first four ingredients (besides sugar, which is usually listed 2nd) in formula are four of the top ten allergens, including peanut oil? (Smith, nd.)

Children with no attachment skills, empathy or sympathy are becoming so dangerous that my fourth grader had to have practice 'lock downs' with her tornado and fire drills. (Karr &Wiley, 1997) In her second grade class, if the timing was off it was impossible to even get into the classroom until the line of kids waiting for their morning Ritalin had been dosed and cleared away. I had home-schooled for a while and people asked me if I wasn't concerned about socialization…what socialization would that be? What she got from the kid who tried to stab her with a pencil? Or, the kid who pushed her face into the pavement on the first day? Or maybe the 'socialization' she got that had her vomiting for days and spiking a temperature of 103 degrees? The child that shared that with her told her mother she didn't feel good as she was dropped off at school and her mother told her 'when you start puking, call me.'

We've lowered the bar on 'normal' so that we can feel good about what can, not should, be expected of our children. Mothers of gently, naturally born, attachment parented, breastfeed babies are often told, "I could never take my kid everywhere! They would drive me nuts!" or "Wow! Your baby is so smart! Good genes!" or "How lucky you are that you get to stay home!" even though luck had nothing to do with it and many personal sacrifices were made to prioritize that option.

Postpartum depression (PPD) got a lot of press after the Yates case, in which a mother murdered her five children due to postpartum psychosis. PPD got some much needed attention, but it wasn't long before it was deemed 'normal' as long as it didn't degrade into psychosis. Why? Because so many women experience it. Is what they experience due to birth, or what has become of birth when all of the natural mechanisms in place for the perpetuation of the species are tampered with?

Finally, some researchers are looking into that and wondering if maybe what American women are experiencing isn't postpartum depression (PPD), but post-traumatic stress disorder (PTSD). (Ayers & Pickering, 2001) Listen to mothers of the typical American birth tell their 'war stories' as they show off their scars and it's an easy leap to make. If the process of birth were the cause, it would stand to reason that other cultures would be experiencing the same rise. That doesn't seem to be the case. Plenty of mothers here and around the world aren't experiencing PPD or PTSD at the rates seen in obstetrically managed mothers in the US.

Granted, this is a disparate grouping of problems. The one thing they all have in common is that their origins may be in the childbearing year, yet the consequences last a lifetime.

It would be ridiculous to insinuate that any one thing is responsible for all of society's ills, yet there is undoubtedly a cumulative effect on health and emotional well-being when brain development is disrupted due to poor nutrition, smoking, drugs (including non-medically indicated labor drugs), lack of brain stimulation and/or lack of mother's milk. The majority of these things also disrupt the bonding process, which leads to other problems in the mother-baby dyad. Thus, mothers begin their new relationship facing challenges they accept as just 'normal' and wonder why they are having a rough time!

Mothers need to know what true 'normal' is and where 'average' lies so they know when to ask for help. They need to know what choices or actions can contribute to 'abnormal' so they can avoid them. Instead infant growth charts are printed by formula companies with 'average' determined by children who have never had a drop of milk that their mother's body made specifically for them! Mothers who do feed their babies human milk are being told their children fall outside of the 'norm!' It doesn't seem to occur to many people to ponder the fact that cows milk is made for baby cows with four stomachs, weighing over 100 pounds at birth. Mothers are instructed not to give babies under 12 months cow's milk because of the allergenic properties, yet most formula is made from, you guessed it, cow's milk. If not cow's milk, soy, which is also on the list of top ten allergens, as well as being of concern due to the phytoestrogens. (Tuohy, 2003)

The corruption of the natural processes meant to ensure the continuation of the species can only go so far. We are only glimpsing the ramifications of our actions. Women who have had, or are having, empowering experiences, who are making choices that bring themselves and their families peace and health, need to pass on their wisdom. This is about fact gathering and basing decisions on solid evidence instead of belief.

It's about judging success by results. How's the current system working?

Folks, this is NOT healthy.

Journal Exploration:

Who will you allow to shape your future?
How might their beliefs color what they experience as real or
    possible?
What are their motivations?
What are their biases? Their beliefs?
Are their beliefs, or yours, based on fact? Personal experience?
    History?
Is it time that some concepts be modified or abandoned in order
    for you to create a better birth experience and smoother
    postpartum transition?
Are you open to the idea that perception is reality?

In other words, is what you're doing working toward your own best birth? If you say the thing you are most afraid of is a cesarean and your doctor insists that you will need one because your baby is breech, do you seek out a caregiver skilled in breech, knowing that a cesarean for breech can more dangerous for the mother with no improvement in outcome for the baby? (Childbirth.org, 1998; Kotaska, Menticoglou, Gagnon, Farine, Basso, Bos, Delisle, Grabowska, Hudon, Mundle, Murphy-Kaulbeck, Ouellet, Pressey, & Roggensack, 2009) Have you sought out and tried any of the known successful techniques for turning a breech to head down? (Mehl, 1994) Why or why not?

If you desire a VBAC and your doctor will only allow it if you have an epidural and augmentation, do you gather the evidence against such dangerous protocol? Do you insist he follow evidence-based practice or let him know you plan to find a provider who will?

Are you happy? Empowered? Healthy? Do you feel confident, knowledgeable and safe? Be honest with yourself. Is every visit a confrontation or exercise in futility? Are you really, truly being heard?

"NO ONE CAN MAKE YOU FEEL INFERIOR WITHOUT YOUR CONSENT." ELEANOR

Are your provider's actions and words saying the same thing? "Oh, we only use intervention when it's necessary" doesn't hold water when you are routinely given every non-medically indicated test in the book.

If coercion is used to manipulate you in pregnancy, why would you expect different at your birth? If intimidation seems second nature, pay attention. A good doctor never says, "Am I the only one that cares about this baby?"

Good doctors react in a reasonable manner to reasonable requests. They appreciate a parent responsible enough to participate in their own good health. They see the wisdom in a good working relationship with actual informed consent. Find those doctors...or a good midwife. Not doing so means that you have agreed to the outcome, good or bad.

A picture paints a thousand words, so let's paint...

A woman comes to an independent childbirth class. She takes everything she is learning to her care provider, expecting to be able to talk about her concerns. Her provider refuses to look at the material from her class, with the comment that it's all garbage because the instructor 'didn't bother to get an education,' showing his ignorance regarding the education and training of autonomous childbirth education certification.

The mother keeps going, keeps pushing for care that is individualized to her. He continues to become more irate with each visit, with each question, until finally, he (fairly) tells her, "If you don't like the way I do things, find another doctor!"

For whatever reason, she doesn't.

Her biggest fear is of episiotomy* and the affect it could have on her life. She shares this with her doctor, who tells her that he will only do it if he has to. He become irritated that she asks how often he finds it's necessary.

His actions become increasingly punitive, yet she keeps going back.

Her birth includes a huge episiotomy that extends into a 4th degree laceration (when the tear extends through the rectum...seen almost exclusively with an episiotomy).

Say the mother wants to blame the doctor for everything gone wrong in her life since the birth by suing the doctor and she asks the childbirth educator to help her.

*episiotomy-a cut made to the vagina to made the opening bigger

If the CBE subscribes to the philosophy of responsible decision-making I'm talking about here, how do you think she would respond to such a request? She would refuse, of course, and remind the mother that she chose the care-provider and the birth location with full knowledge of the probabilities.

Alternatively, if you accept such treatment and find yourself saying, "It's the price you pay for a good doctor" take that as your cue to take responsibility for your situation...and then find a new doctor. Good doctors charge paper money for office visits—they don't demand pieces of your broken soul or abused body. You deserve better. Your baby deserves better. Husbands, your wives...the mothers of your children...deserve the best. You change a situation like those above. Situations like it happen so often only because they can. You DO have the power to change it.

Good physicians know all this is true and try to provide safe and effective care. They have formed groups like 'Physicians for Midwives' in many states, and the peer pressure they face is incredible. They will be the first to tell you that good care does not mean bad treatment. That's why this book is so important...it helps you spot the good guys.

CHAPTER 2
Birth Beliefs

It's easy to identify the women who've taken special care to do their birthing and parenting research.

No two parenting approaches may be the same, but those who've done the work are enjoying the path of parenting, whatever has befallen them along the way. They are informed and confident in their decisions. These mothers can't wait to tell you about their incredible labors, drug free, ecstatic, pain free, or at least manageable births. They are so blissful they seem almost evangelical in their zeal to share the joys of motherhood, even if Mother Nature tosses them a few challenges. Because they have more good days than bad, these challenges are met head on and probably soon forgotten. They forgive themselves when they mess up.

So why do so many mothers feel ripped off, assuming the joyful mothers aren't for real, that such an ideal doesn't exist? Why are some mothers angry and bitter? It might be because they believe great births exist, but believe they can't have them, as illustrated by the following mother, reviewing Naomi Wolf's book, *Misconceptions: Truth, Lies and the Unexpected on the Journey to Motherhood*:

"…all the happy-earth-mama books about midwifery and doulas and all those candlelit bonding moments with a new squealing infant are put in their place---as happy fairytales that happen to a few women in America." (Siciliano, 2009)

The irony is, it happens to so few women because so few women make the choices that result in those births…not because they aren't possible! The 'fairy tale' births could be the norm!

The women who have been 'lucky' enough to have safe and satisfying births (although I might argue luck was a small contribution) are women with imperfect lives—nobody is perfect—but they educate themselves, they have a support system and they operate from a place of empowerment. Their convictions are strong because they are sure they are doing what works for themselves and their babies. Certainly there are parents who do all this and more who find themselves in situations they would not choose. However, in determining the most significant factors in controlling what can be controlled, education and support are key.

These happy mothers, because they want others to be able to enjoy the journey as much as they do, are often accused of trying to make other mothers 'guilty' for making different choices, when what they are trying to do is share the choices that brought them joy. Of course, in any population there will be a few judgmental people, but in my experience, most of the time, it's not the happy parent that is doing the judging, but the unhappy parent. The happy parent's only mistake is assuming that when women say they want a less traumatic birth next time, they really mean it. Knowing that drama and chaos and sadness can almost always be avoided in birth, they give advice they thought was solicited. Then they are puzzled by the 'yeah, buts…' that follow.

Naomi Wolf, in *Misconceptions*, doubts the existence of these happy moms who face few challenges in their new role. (Note that I did not say 'no challenges.') While her book is an excellent read with invaluable information, and I respect her very much, she draws some interesting conclusions that I didn't expect from such a smart woman.

Pages and pages are devoted to exposing the detriments of the current system and praising the possibilities if we were to adopt something closer to the midwifery model of care. She concedes that home birth is as safe or safer than hospital and backs it up. She also concedes that VBAC is preferable to repeat cesarean. Being a mother who seems to have felt cheated by the system the first time around, she does make somewhat different choices with her second baby. Her reasoning for not having the home birth that she admits might have had a different outcome? Birth is so excruciating (another belief that pervades the book is that this must be so without the aid of drugs) that if she wants an epidural she can't have one at home. True. She can't. Why? Because it carries such risks that they can't be dealt with at home!

However, that's not the part that left me confused. If a woman is laboring at home with a qualified midwife or competent doctor and there is a complication or she decides she just can't manage without an epidural, she's free to get up and go to the hospital for any assistance she may need. The odds are that at home neither she nor her baby will need medical assistance or experience the sort of pain that she felt in the hospital the first time. (Mehl, Peterson, Shaw, & Creavy, 1978)

If she does, there's no reason she can't go to the hospital. However, I'd like to see a women in active labor at the hospital declare that she's feeling good and wants to go home to push her baby out!

At first glance, the reasoning behind a 'just in case' philosophy seems logical, but it stems from a faulty belief, which makes it illogical. I admire Naomi Wolf immensely. She's written a scathing expose' on American obstetrical care that's cuttingly witty and strong on data. She used her disillusionment with her first birth to write a book about how many women are dissatisfied with their experience. She seems to get it, at least on paper. Yet, it seems to me she makes many faulty assumptions apparently based on fear...fear of pain being primary. Words and actions diverge greatly here and this seems so inconsistent. But the nature of the fear is typically subconscious, allowing many women to coast through pregnancy without questioning much because, after all, they feel fine and they aren't scared. Some women will freely admit they are terrified, but many more fall into the 'see no evil' category.

Illustrating that Wolf is probably quite typical in her thinking is that her book is heavy on blame and it seems to me, short on responsibility. At one point, she blames hospital childbirth class and the books she read for not being truthful. She contends they misled her into making bad choices. She admits that there are independent childbirth classes that do give more useful information (though natural birth advocates are called 'ideological naturalists' who 'romanticize the pain'). She quotes several books out there that actually do give solid strategic planning advice, just as there are caregivers available that have proven to have better outcomes. Resources that she researched...after her births. During her pregnancy she didn't seek out those classes or use the information in the books.

She's angry that the classes she chose didn't tell her the 'truth.' Would she have wanted to hear the documented risks of epidurals? Because of her fear of pain and disbelieve of the idea that pain can be comfortable without drugs, likely not. However, it's a moot point, because her hospital class very probably could not have given her that information. I know when I was a childbirth educator at one hospital I was not free to share say anything that contradicted what friendly visiting anesthesiologist said, even if I could offer independent scientific studies. He, however, could cite studies supporting non-medical use of medications conducted by anesthesiologists and funded by drug companies!

Hm...no conflict of interest here. For a childbirth educator to even let on that she possesses such information is cause for termination. Why? Remember who signs her check? When you are low man on the totem pole it isn't wise to expose the great and powerful Oz. I'm not being cynical, I'm being brutally honest. I've been there, I know. I have also been fortunate enough to teach in a hospital where evidence and result-based success is valued, so I know those exist as well. However, they are a rarity. Even in those institutions, the teacher must teach what the parents want to learn or the seats will sit empty. Sadly, many parents take a class to hear the wonders of drugs, not the risks, and to become familiar with the hospital layout and protocols. For childbirth educators went into the profession to help women have safer, more comfortable births it's very frustrating to be relegated to tour guide and drug pusher.

64

Admittedly safer, more empowering options are dismissed for a variety of reasons. The longer I do this, the more I understand just how many reasons. I contend beliefs and fears about birth cause women to reject ideas that could be of use to them. Yet, I admit that I have a hard time understanding why a childbirth educator teaching natural childbirth techniques that often result in comfortable birth is accused of 'lying' when she can demonstrate efficacy! When a class includes testimonials and video of more comfortable, painless or even orgasmic birth, why don't more women find this intriguing?

> "IT'S EASIER TO BE NICE THAN TO BE HONEST, BUT IT'S MORE IMPORTANT TO BE RESPECTED THAN TO BE LIKED."
> (ELI WIESEL)

Thousands of women are giving birth quickly and painlessly though Mongan Method HypnoBirthing®, thousands more are doing the same spontaneously. Some women even give birth orgasmically. Because Wolf doesn't believe it can be anything other that what she experienced...and what her friends have experienced...she insists painless birth can't possibly be true.

Still and all, though Wolf opted for surgery for her second birth, she was empowered by the decision. That makes all the difference. For in the end, it doesn't matter what other people think...only that she made her own best decision.

It's those women who don't make their decisions from a place of knowledge, or who don't recognize that they are making decisions at all, that end up with regret. They go along with whatever they are told 'every body' does (or has to do) not realizing that by not making choices, they are still choosing. But they are doing so with an unspoken fear that 'something' will go wrong. Or they may fear of how they might look to others if they do something different. Perhaps they even fear that they'll make a wrong decision, and if someone else makes the decisions for them, someone else will be to blame if something goes wrong.

It is my assertion that ultimately these types of non-decisions are based on some kind of fear. Perhaps even, as suggested in *Flight from Death: The Quest for Immortality* (Transcendental Media, 2003) it is the universal fear of death. They operate from a 'just in case' mentality, yet they have no firm idea of what the actual possibility of 'just in case' is. When I was pregnant and people learned I was having a planned home birth with a midwife they would exclaim in alarm, "What if something happens?!" I'd ask, "Like what?"

More than one person responded, "What if the cord is wrapped around the neck and it chokes the baby?" as if I was an idiot for not considering that.

I'd take the opportunity to explain that 30% of the time, there is a loop of cord around the baby's neck. It's a variation of normal, not a complication. (There actually was with my baby.) Midwives will either un-loop it over the baby's head, loosen it so that the baby can be born through the loop or 'somersault' the baby through. No big deal. A baby is not breathing through his or her windpipe, thus it is impossible for the baby to be 'choked' by the umbilical cord. However, very rarely the cord will be very short or wrapped more than once restricting blood flow through the cord, and midwives are trained to recognize such an event and have the tools and skills to manage such a situation at home.

Of course, it just sounds prudent to approach birth 'proactively'... except that the 'proactive' approach currently in use isn't working. More mothers and babies are dying than 20 years ago, when fewer interventions were used. More mothers and babies are dying because of the technology than natural birth complications.

Parents don't realize (or won't admit) that fear is actually the motivating force behind their decisions. Most of the time my request for specific 'what ifs' are met with either stunned silence because they can't come up with something, or the story of their own birth with some tragic complication. A large percentage of the time, said complication was iatrogenic (doctor caused) or nosocomial (hospital caused)...not common in natural (and what should be 'normal') birth. Fear of the unknown is at the bottom of it all...irrational fear not substantiated by fact.

Those that don't get it are the 'blamers'. They blame doctors for not giving them the perfect experience or the perfect child. It's someone else's fault when bad things happen. Someone always has to pay for their misfortune. These people drive the malpractice rates up and create the current environment in which defensive medicine thrives...creating the vicious cycle of overused and abused technology.

Fear rules these people. They insist pregnancy and birth are rift with calamity. This fear has permeated the caring professionals within the broken system. It translates into fear of litigation. Obstetricians aren't being mean...they are very afraid! According to the World Health Organization, at least half of all cesareans (at least 500,000 a year in 2003) are unnecessary and it all comes back to fear.

Fearful parents will torture themselves with guilt, second-guess themselves at every turn...and then make the same decisions again, and again. This reinforces their belief that birth is dangerous because choosing the same actions results in the same consequences. They may spiral into severe PPD or even PTSD, all the while demanding to know 'why me?' When discussions of birth come up (as they invariably do when women gather) women who have done their homework will sometimes be able to see 'why,' but they will be hesitant to volunteer what they know, lest they be labeled 'judgmental.' If someone points out that there might have bee a multitude of choices that, by virtue of commonsense and evidence, might have netted a different outcome, it isn't seen as helpful. It's seen as blaming the victim.

To break out of this vicious cycle, we have to challenge what we know that isn't really so about the current maternity care system in the US. How effective is it at improving the lives of mothers and babies? It would seem not very as we have seen. What perpetuates it? Are there better alternatives to the choices that 'everybody else' makes? Failing to investigate these questions means you can't possibly make educated choices.

If you don't know this stuff you are operating without the necessary information and skills to create the results you want.

I hear examples of unintentionally created results so often I can finish a mother's story before she does. I'm not psychic, it's just that predictable.

For instance, a woman goes in for 'her' (because it's 'standard of care' it's just part of this right of passage deserving of a personal pronoun) gestational diabetes test. She's labeled with Gestational Diabetes and put on a low salt, low calorie, and yes low-sugar, restricted diet. This diet leads to pre-eclampsia, a pregnancy complication which is a reason for an emergency cesarean, but might have been avoided in the first place through proper nutrition. (Brewer, 1985)

The shortcomings of this particular test were presented in the last chapter. None-the-less, it is standard of care that often leads questionable treatment, which even more often leads to unnecessary surgery.

Another example: A woman, laboring quite nicely, is 'too comfortable.' Her caregiver is afraid that her labor has petered out since she looks too calm and relaxed. He suggests that they break her water to 'speed things up.'

She doesn't know that studies show no significant difference in length of labor (Rosen & Peisner, 1983; Seitchik, Holden & Castillio, 1985.) with amniotomy (breaking the water). She doesn't know that if a baby is high in the pelvis when water is artificially ruptured, there is a high likelihood that her baby will drop down in an unfavorable position. The fancy term is 'transverse arrest,' which basically means the baby is stuck.

This is a situation that was created, not encountered. (Fraser et al, 1993)

Amniotomy also accounts for the largest portion of cesareans for infection, failure to progress and cord prolapse (when the cord is washed down with the tide of water ahead of the baby...remember, the baby gets oxygen from the cord). (Kariniemi, 1983; Levy et al, 1984; Goer, 1995) Ask ten women to tell you about their births and nearly all of them will contain the words "...and then they broke my water." Interesting terminology, instead of "...and then I let them break my water" considering this action requires someone's fingers having access to the mother's vagina. Women do not sacrifice their autonomy just because they are pregnant or in labor. They have a right to informed consent and the right to refuse routine interventions.

"Birth" is blamed for these frightening situations. We don't have such high cesarean rates, or some of the worst mortality and morbidity rates, in the developed world because birth is dangerous, but because obstetrically managed birth is. Countries with better outcomes know better than to have surgical specialist dealing in pathology care for healthy women for a normal physiological process.

The idea of surgical specialists being the preferred caregiver for a normal, physiological process is analogous to a cardiovascular surgeon doing all routine exams on men over 50 or orthopedic surgeons for skinned knees!

Sure it sounds ridiculous, unless it were introduced the way obstetrics was, over 80 years, with powerful spin-doctors.

After all, a fall bad enough to break the skin could cause a broken bone. Sometimes falls in the elderly require specialist care because their bones are brittle, and the very young because their bones are still growing. If it's good for them, think how we can help everyone else!

Some people would resist, of course. Then word would get out that those seeing specialists got strong pharmacological pain relief!

A sprain hurts really badly, even if it's not a break...but without going to the specialist, one can't get the drugs...and gee, maybe there could be something worse wrong.

It might not even take 80 years for people to start imagining that there is no safe fall to handle at home. Bandages would seem primitive. "You didn't take your kid to the doctor for that banged-up knee?! Don't you want the best for him? What if there is something wrong you can't see just by looking! You know, my nephew would have died if he hadn't been in the hospital after his skiing accident! He thought it was just a sprain, but good thing he went because he almost bled to death during the knee replacement!"

This is essentially how the normalcy of birth turned into a medical event.

Fear of birth, and fear of pain in birth, has created such panic that women prefer elective paraplegia to being an active participant in the most amazing event in their lives. They submit unquestioningly to rituals with no basis in reality. Statistically, they have a better chance of dying on the way to the hospital (20 in 100,000 for car accidents in women of childbearing age) than they do during a normal, natural birth (6 in 100,000) yet IVs aren't standard issue in cars. Of course, if they are one of the 1 in 3 women who will get a cesarean their odds of dying are highest of all, 35 in 100,000.

As for pain, there are plenty of women giving birth comfortably, even painlessly, so it is possible to do it without drugs and there are ways to learn how.

Where does the fear that allows this madness to continue come from? Is it misinformation or lack of information? Is it that we've given up making decisions for ourselves altogether?

70

1.) If you look into the future at the possible and probable consequences to you, your family and your baby for this choice, what do you see? Could you live with the worse case scenario with a clear conscience?

2.) If someone chooses differently, how does that make you feel?

3.) Is this choice in the best interest of your baby? How do you know? How much do you know about the ramifications of both of (or all of) your options? What does common sense logic tell you? Intuition? Science?

4.) If there is a doubt about whether this decision is in the best interest of your child, what have you done to make a better choice more attainable?

5.) What sacrifice is being asked of you? Do you make it for your child willingly? How does it compare for the sacrifice your baby is being asked to make? If your child were able to speak, what do you think he or she would choose? Why?

6.) In a perfect world, would this be your choice? If not, why? What can you do to make it perfect enough for this choice to happen?

7.) If you are aware that there is an option that is better and/or safer for your baby in the short or long term, why do you choose not to consider it? It is because you can't or because you won't?

8.) Is this choice irreversible?

9.) Is this a life decision? Does it enhance or contaminate your relationship with your baby? Is it a positive or negative contribution to your baby's health? Do you like yourself for making it?

10.) Do you feel the need to make excuses or defend your choice?

11.) Does this act tell your baby, "I love you"? Does it show your baby or child that you love him or her above all else?

12.) If your baby could speak, would you make this same decision? Would you want someone to make this decision for you if you were unable to communicate your wishes? If your life were recorded, would you do the same?

13.) Would your actions be any different toward an adult that you love if they were helpless and totally dependent on you? Does your baby deserve at least that much?

Please bear in mind as you read examples of how choices in the childbearing year have gone awry, that I speak in generalities, though I use specific, real-life examples. I am using the most common stories I hear, so they may very well seem familiar. They are what has become 'the norm.'

No matter what choices you make, they are yours to make. If you want every intervention, useful, dangerous or just plain nonsensical, go for it. Just know what the consequences of your actions are so you can own them when the inevitable happens. If somehow you cheat the statistics, great. At least you will have made your decisions consciously and with purposeful intent.

My primary goal is to help women have safer births that are unique, rewarding and dignified, if that's what they want. Somehow, women have gotten the idea that safety and emotionally satisfying are mutually exclusive in birth, which is patently false.

You don't need to give up your power and autonomy to have a safe birth. There are cause and effect relationships every step of the way to motherhood that influence the experience. Knowledge makes you the one in control, which is where you need to be. You are the one that will live with the consequences of your actions — or non-actions as the case may be.

In the case of your care provider choice, you sign the check, either directly or through a proxy in the form of your insurance provider. Your caregiver works for you. You have the right, and the responsibility, not to be a passive in this relationship. If your insurance company is owned by doctors, it still comes down to you and how hard you are willing to fight for the safety of your baby. No one said this journey would be an easy one to navigate, but it is the most important you'll ever embark upon. As you research the multitude of decisions and weigh the risk/benefit ratio, some seem clear cut; others, not so much. Just remember that no one should invest what they can't afford to lose. In this case, the investment is your baby's life.

Will you trust that to luck and bad information or will you dig deeper? Do you feel comfortable being a partner in our own care?

Dr. Phil has several works that stress that a healthy relationship must meet the needs of both people. This is a universal truth that applies to more than just your primary love relationship. It applies to your relationship with your care provider and later to the mother-baby relationship. So many women get so little time with their provider that they feel they can't ask questions. That is unacceptable when the stakes are this high.

In the US we are not taught to take responsibility for ourselves or the condition of our relationships. We are not taught how to parent. We are not encouraged to question authority. We assume our care providers always have a good reason for doing what they do and that it's for our own good. We tend to do what our own parents did or what our friends do, assuming there is a good reason they do what they do. Unfortunately, that's not always the case.

This reminds me of a story I read once about a young woman making her first holiday ham. When her husband saw her cut the ends off the ham, he asked her why she did that. She pondered a moment and replied, "I don't know. That's just how my mom always did it."

She called her mother to ask her what the purpose was in cutting off the ends of the ham. Her mother told her she wasn't really sure why...it was just how her mother did it.

So the mother called the grandmother and asked, "Why do you cut the ends off the ham? Does it make it juicier? Does it cook faster?"

"Not that I know of." replied the grandmother. "I always do it because the ham never fits in my pan!"

There was a time when an elite few held all information. In my mother's day, it wasn't an easy feat to compare and contrast the

73

incoming data, what little of it there was. Today, books like *The Thinking Woman's Guide to Better Birth* and *Obstetrical Myths versus Research Realities* should be on every pregnant woman's coffee table.

They aren't, not because they aren't useful, but they don't tell women what they want to hear. They only tell the truth.

My mother's generation should feel good about doing the best they could with what they had. They should not feel it's an indictment of their choices if their daughters know more and do better. And in this day of instant information, there is no reason not to know better.

We spend four to twelve years in college learning to do a job that may last 40 years if we're lucky. We will hold a position that, when we leave, will be filled by someone new in a matter of days.

We will work with people who, for the most part, know nothing of our hopes, dreams or fears even though we will spend more time with them than our own children.

Yet, I have parents from my classes complain that eight hours of childbirth preparation classes takes up too much of their time. Parents are parents for life. Mothers hold generations within them. Your children will never forget you and cannot replace you. Through them, you either make the world a little better...or a little more scary. It's my own personal opinion that three semesters of 'Parenting' ought to be a mandatory in every high school diploma or college degree.

This is a crash course in responsible parenting. You must be willing to gather data every day staring right now. Make a commitment to your baby and yourself because there are no 'do-overs'. You get one chance to grow this baby the body it will inhabit for a lifetime. You may only get to experience birth once or twice in your life. Make those memories precious.

In 50 years do you want to be swapping birth stories filled with regret with your bridge club, or will you be misty eyed with joy as you pass empowerment on to your granddaughter?

Talk to elderly women in nursing homes. Ask them which they remember better, the births of their children or the amounts of their bonuses? Do they recall their first promotion with the same sweet sadness as the first time their nursling gave them a milky smile?

Sure, there are women who thrive on the accolades of the competitive business world. More power to 'em! I'm all for women's empowerment in all forms. I believe in having it all, maybe just not all having it all at the same time.

However, if you are reading this book because you are pregnant, make every effort count. You won't get another chance to shape your baby's life in such a profound way.

People can spend more time shopping for a car or home than they put into their births. They sacrifice years and thousands of dollars to go to college while they live on boxed macaroni and cheese, but balk at the investment of a couple of years of love and maybe some penny pinching during their children's most important developmental years.

Whether you've looked at mothers and thought "I hope it's that easy for me!" or "Boy, is she lucky she can stay home." Or, even "What a brat that kid is!" know that coincidence and luck play a very small part. Ask the mothers who loved giving birth, and love being a mom why they do what they do. Ask mothers who like to be around their kids, and who's kids you like to be around what they did or didn't do and why. Then emulate their success.

Journal exploration:

What do I want to avoid during my pregnancy and birth? Is it conceivable that it is within my power to avoid this/these?

What have I done to ensure (where possible) the things I want or avoid the things I don't?

Can I accept that I may have to examine some of my choices or gather more information?

Am I communicating my needs clearly to my care-provider and partner?

Do I find myself justifying inconsistency in my provider's words and actions?

Do I continue to trust when maybe I should question?

Am I standing up for my parental rights and asking for what I need?

Am I treating myself with the dignity & respect a mother deserves? Am I requiring it of others? Am I insisting my baby be treated with respect?

Am I realistic in my pregnancy, birth and parenting expectations?

CHAPTER 3
Mother Guilt

I will not cheat you out of your empowerment by telling you what is comfortable, instead of what you need to know. Too many books out there are telling you what to expect, but so few are telling you that you should expect more.

I believe it's time to be honest about some of our collective sacred cows. We have been politically correct about so many things for so long that we've lost sight of common sense. Many women come to their transition into motherhood confused and afraid instead of strong and excited to be a part of the Mystery. Many spend their lives feeling guilty for what they could not control, others, conversely, abdicating responsibility for their decisions.

Discussion of mothering has become as taboo as discussing religion or politics. Women have so many 'choices' now that to suggest one choice is better for babies than another is to risk offense. We tiptoe around certain things under the guise of 'being sensitive.'

What has happened is that in our attempt to be sensitive to mothers who can't make the choices they know are best for their babies, we have made all options seem equal when in reality they simply aren't.

The problem with this is two-fold. First-of-all, it doesn't shield the mother who is truly unable to give her child what she knows is best. What it does do is put women who can but won't in the same category, providing an excuse to take the path of least resistance instead of putting the best interest of the child first. The courts use the willingness of a custodial or adoptive parent to put 'the best interest of the child first' as a measure of good parenting. Examples abound of natural parents not being held to the same standard.

There are women who've lost their breasts to cancer who have little patience with women who have perfectly functioning breasts who refuse to feed their baby the milk made specifically for him because they say they 'can't' when they really mean 'I don't want to.'

There are single mothers, with no support system, who cry every morning when they have to leave their child with an allomother*, working two jobs and going to school with their only reward watching their child sleep in the moonlight with the hope that their hard work will eventually allow them to spend time with their child when he's awake.

What might they be thinking when they hear a fellow working mother say she works because she couldn't stand to be with her whining, teething baby…a baby obviously in need of mothering. (I am not talking here of a mother who has just had enough for that day or that week and needs a break, as all mothers do, but of a 'mother' who dislikes the very act of mothering.)

Consider the woman who has eagerly anticipated her labor and birth as rite-of-passage but must have a cesarean due to cord prolapse or some other real medical indication. Grateful for the surgery that saved her child's life, or her own, she still grieves the loss of her dream. When she hears about a woman who could have birthed naturally, but instead chose surgery for something as trivial as knowing the birth date in advance to plan around it, it would be understandable if she were confused by such a choice. The surgery that is used with medical indication to save a life is the same surgery that carries a four times greater mortality (death) rate when it's done in the absence of a medical reason. How can anyone seriously say that to point this out is in any way, shape, or form a disservice to the woman did what she had to do to save her child?

*Allomother is a term used in Mother Nature: A History of Mothers, Infants, and Natural Selection by Sarah Blaffer Hrdy, Pantheon Books, 1999 in reference to mother substitutes.

To put these mothers all in the same category isn't fair. To suggest that fathers (or co-parents) are superfluous, or that it doesn't matter whether a mother or substitute mother raises their baby, or that the stay at home mother is 'lucky' is an insult.

Are there 'stay-at-home' mothers who don't actually mother at all? Of course. Are there very loving corporate mothers who are able to organize their time so that their baby never has an allomother? Naturally. Are there mothers who are the primary bread winners or who have functional insurance through work that the family needs, who go to extraordinary measures to ensure that even though the situation isn't their ideal, it has minimal impact on their children? Absolutely. Remember...no all or nothing thinking. There are always exceptions to the rule.

However, the way that this wide range of parental personal philosophy is dealt with is that it isn't. Certain topics are approached with prefaced with 'Of course it's a mother's choice, but...' or not considered at all. Does that mean anyone has the right to judge anyone for making different choices than themselves?

They don't have the right because they don't have the power. No one can know what's best for your child, in your circumstance. We know what the evidence says is probably best for most children in most circumstances. We know what's possible for most moms when they are determined to do their best. Only you know what is best for you. If you've made your decisions with the best of intent, there is no need for the self-imposed emotion of guilt.

Yes, a self-imposed emotion. No one can make you feel guilty unless you agree to feel it. The purpose of guilt is that it guides us to aspire to "do the best we can with what we have, and when we know better we do better" (Maya Angelou). We must learn to distinguish true guilt as a message from our conscience from the useless punishment we heap on ourselves mistakenly labeled as guilt. Language often reveals the difference. Using the breastfeeding analogy again, an adoptive mother does not apologize for bottle-feeding her infant. She has no reason to and she knows it. (I know that someone will write to tell me that some adoptive mothers are able to breast feed. I am aware of that, but not all, and even those who do probably won't do so exclusively. Artificial baby milk originated out of orphaned baby situations so it's a valid analogy.) A mother who made the choice not to breastfeed is likely to say "I really wanted to breastfeed, but..." Anytime "but" is in a sentence, everything that comes before is negated for what comes after it. Try it. Ok, now reverse it. Have you ever heard a breastfeeding mother ever say "I really wanted to formula feed, but..."

At least a woman who says, "I know that the milk from my own body is the best for my baby that grew in my body. I still didn't want to breastfeed." is being honest. Even if one disagrees with the intent behind the decision, you can respect that she'd have the bold ovaries to stand up to it. A mother that is defensive or makes excuses does a fine job of judging herself. Of course, often that is externalized so her perception will be that others are judging her, but that doesn't change that it really is a reflection of what she knows in her heart.

I can speak on this subject of mother-guilt with certainty because as a mother I have had nearly every single action I've taken on behalf of my child, from birthing at home, to vegetarianism, to my spiritual path, questioned and judged, sometimes quite vocally and with great hostility. I feel no guilt for my choices, even when they are different from most of the people I know. I am confident that I had the information I needed to make the best choices for my child and hold dear my right to do so. I can count on one hand the number of times that I have felt even a moment of regret when information came to light that might have altered a past course of action. In that moment, I had a couple of options. I could feel guilt and punish myself indefinitely, but make the same choices I've made in the past, or I could use the new information to make a different choice, forgiving myself for the past that I cannot change. I chose the latter.

I share this information with compassion and the best intent. I have no control over how the facts are received or perceived. I share it because of the many mothers who have regrets these days. Things they wish they knew then that they know now.

Like the mother who smoked like a chimney, as did her husband, who got defensive during class when smoking was discussed. The parents who didn't want to hear about the effects of smoking on pregnancy, birth and babies. The parents who didn't appreciate people 'making them feel guilty' for their choice to smoke, insisting it's no one's business to judge their lifestyle. The very same parents who lost their baby to SIDS, and upon researching 'why' as part of their healing, found that smoking parents are much more likely to lose babies to SIDS (only one among many issues regarding smoking mothers). The parents who wanted to know 'Why didn't anyone tell us!" instead of "Why didn't I listen?" As a mother, defensiveness and avoidance of information that evokes feelings of guilt can be deadly.

The mom did choose to stop smoking eventually. She was a good mom...just a mom who paid a terrible price for not being able to look at a hard truth. Hindsight is always 20/20.

There are too many women living with the 'what ifs.' The stakes are too high to be worried about egos. This book is not about 'you should'. It asks 'should you'? It gives you 'the rest of the story' and demands that you compare, contrast, and check in with your own heart. Granted, this carries a certain amount of courage, and it demands that we take back responsibility for our own choices. Our children deserve no less.

Journal Exploration:

If you have felt like someone else was in control of your pregnancy up until now, take some time to re-evaluate accountability. To determine this, listen to how you talk about your options: 'Then they did...' or 'Then I had to...'

Thinking back through your pregnancy to date, or to past pregnancies, can you list times when you felt mistreated, ignored, not dealt with fairly and compassionately, made to feel incompetent or defective?

Now go back to each instance, identifying how your action or inaction contributed to the result that made you feel victimized. Were there warning signs? Intuition?

How does one know what is 'right'? The answer lies inside you, with your conscience and that 'wiggly' feeling in your stomach, as my daughter calls it. However, if following your intuition and your body's innate wisdom is a new concept, ask yourself the following questions when you are faced with making a decision that will affect both yourself and your child.

Choosing a Care Provider for Your Pregnancy and Birth

At the first sign of pregnancy, many women automatically make an appointment with their primary care physician or obstetrician. Some, aware that the birthing philosophy of their OB/GYN is different than their own, or who realize that adequate well-woman care does not necessarily translate into good maternity care, will seek out a different doctor for their pregnancy and birth.

Individual circumstance and personal preference play a large role in whether parents will look outside of their geographical area, or if the experiences of friends and family members influence their choice of provider.

In other cases, fear is a silent participant in the process of selection. Fathers-to-be rarely give a second thought to who will care for the love-of-their-life at her most vulnerable time. At this stage of the game, it's still in the realm of 'women's business' that they've never been involved in before. Before now, it's never been about who will be the first person to meet their child who is very much an abstract at this point.

"THOSE WHO DO NOT LEARN FROM THE PAST ARE DESTINED TO REPEAT IT."
WINSTON CHURCHILL

Early pregnancy is a very emotional time. Even if the pregnancy has been planned for, or possibly orchestrated with intensive reproductive technology, there may be a moment or two of ambivalence...a feeling of "Oh no! What was I thinking?!" With unplanned pregnancies, there may be a sense of panic or fear. In any scenario, there is a sense of the world shifting with the emotional enormity of how life will change. Sometimes, it's a confusing, emotional feeling that begs for stability and familiarity to balance the excitement and the mysterious unknown.

The fierce protectiveness of mother-love hasn't usually kicked in. Mom doesn't necessarily feel any different physically just yet. Because she feels so 'normal,' it may seem quite logical to make the call to someone who's been part of her 'normal' life. It may be the wise choice...or it may not.

This first choice as a parent may make the difference between life and death for you or your baby. Sound dramatic? It is. The sad part is that American mothers aren't even aware that they have choices to make, much less that their empowerment in making those choices could very well change the direction of the rest of their lives.

Knowledge is power. How well do you know your doctor? Do you know his/her cesarean rate? Do you know the infant mortality (death) rate for your state? For your county? For your hospital? Do you know what routine practices your doctor has as part of his standard protocol? Do you know if those practices are supported as safe and effective by scientific evidence? Does it sound overwhelming that one should even have to consider all this stuff?

Again, it is. However, it's very important. It's not as intimidating to gather this data as it sounds, for the most part. It may take a couple of hours to look up the information for your region on the internet. Consider it a small investment in the safety of your child.

Start out with the big picture and narrow the field. Begin at the national level so you have the ability to compare your state's outcomes with others. Find the current international statistics. You'll find for yourself that plenty of other countries have few mothers and babies die than the US and that at least 25% of the baby deaths in the US are preventable. The recommendations from The World Health Organization for improving outcomes include...choice of caregiver.

Then look up US infant mortality rates with the Centers for Disease Control (CDC). In 2003 for vaginal birth it's 5.7 per 1,000 births for white babies. For African-American babies, the rate is 14.1 per 1,000.

Next, look for state statistics to determine state, then county mortality rates. The World Heath Organization recommends a 12-15% cesarean rate for optimum outcomes (the most live babies and mothers). Once the rates rise above that rate, the balance of this life-saving technique of last resort shifts so that more lives are lost than saved...hence at least a few preventable deaths. Statistics from countries with the best outcomes bear this out, as do statistics of midwifery communities where cesarean rates are kept low.

What might this information tell you?

Since we know that more African-American babies die than white, usually born to inner-city mothers with few resources and many challenges, we would expect to find that the counties with bigger cities including this population to have higher mortality rates.

Finally, some counties have many hospitals, others just one. In order to utilize the information you've gathered, there must be some small amount of familiarity with your own county resources and population. Once these things are considered, we are left with an educated guess that must be weighed along with the information gathered at the personal level.

Check into cesarean rates, which are an indicator of appropriate birth technology. You could simply ask your doctor or midwife for his or her rate. Because individual doctors and hospitals are not required to divulge mortality, morbidity (injury) or cesarean rates, patients may not get the answers they seek, but there are other sources.* Doctors and hospitals with low rates are very proud of that accomplishment, so if you can't get the data, you actually are getting some very important information.

*See 'Web Resources'

Journal Exploration:

What negative tapes (thoughts that run unbidden through your head) do you have about birth? List the top ten and choose to stop sabotaging yourself now. For each negative comment, think of a positive affirmation using positive language. Focus on what you want, rather than what you don't.

For example:

Negative tape: I don't even want to think about the pain in labor!
    Affirmation: My body is perfectly designed to give birth.
Negative tape: I can't do this!
    Affirmation: I have all the resources I need to give birth gently.
Negative tape: I can't ask my doctor that! He'll think I don't trust him!
    Affirmation: It's good parenting to be assertive in seeking the best care for my baby.*

1.

2.

3.

4.

5.

6.

7.

8.

9.

10.

*Mongan Method HypnoBirthing® taped affirmations are available through practitioners teaching HypnoBirthing classes as well from the HypnoBirthing Institute.

In a large community, sorting this out may require help from organizations existing solely for the purpose of helping mothers make wise choices. Groups of other mothers like Le LeLeche League (a breastfeeding support group) or ICAN (a cesarean awareness group) can be valuable resources. Friends and family are another. Just listen carefully to what they really say. If most of them have had the same doctor and they all rave about him, but most of them have had cesareans, episiotomies, postpartum depression that seems to border on post-traumatic stress disorder, sick babies, premature births or some other catastrophe or another, there's a problem. Birth just doesn't carry that much risk!

If it does with that particular health provider, there's something wrong with that picture. You've already read the mortality rate for vaginal birth and for car accidents for women of childbearing age. If a particular automotive company's cars were involved in far more than the statistical average of deaths, most people would refuse to buy cars from them...even if they came equipped with standard issue IV bags.

Dawn's story illustrates just how difficult it can be to make fact-based decisions in the childbearing year, even if you think you are being dealt with in a fair manner. Her doctor was honest with her. When she asked what his cesarean rate was he replied he did, "quite a few" cesareans. But she liked him. "He sits by the bed with his hand on your belly" she explained. He also used inappropriate and dangerous technology routinely when some of the other doctors in his hospital had abandoned them for more evidence-based care. When she asked about this, he promised that even if he disagreed with her, it was her birth and he'd only use interventions if he had to. He 'had to' a lot.

One of these interventions was routine episiotomy. Her postpartum period was a nightmare. Feeding the baby was hard because I was just in too much pain to get comfortable, and forget sex!

The pain lasted for months. Her husband tried to be patient, but he couldn't understand that even sitting and walking hurt long after the cut healed. She justified the pain she suffered, defending her doctor by saying "Well, I guess that's the price you pay for a good doctor."

Good providers charge standard currency for good care...not body integrity or first-born child. This doctor came highly recommended by friends who also found justifications for his actions instead of questioning his them. His words reassured her all along the way, but his actions were always contrary to his words. He said he believed that pregnancy and birth were natural events, yet test after non-medically indicated test was ordered. He said he believed birth was safe, yet 'just-in-case' technology was employed, revealing his real fears.

EACH PREGNANCY CHOICE LEADS TO THE ONE-AND-ONLY BIRTH OF YOUR CHILD.

Another example of how important it is to pay attention to non-verbal cues and intuition is Phoebe. Her doctor was very personable. She searched long and hard using many of the methods here. She and her husband were smart, savvy parents who weren't willing to settle for second best. Once they found the doctor they liked, subtle changes started to take place. Where they had been told that this doctor believed in minimal technology in the absence of medical indication, new tests were ordered at every visit. Being an informed consumer, Phoebe did her homework.

Often she would find that a test was either not medically necessary or that it was useless...not accurate or developed for women with illnesses she did not have. She would bring in the information. Faced with evidence contrary to his practice, he'd get angry. Phoebe and Ted would leave feeling stressed, often Phoebe in tears and coerced into taking yet another test.

Still they went back. At each visit, he'd try to tell her she was sick. She did the research and knew she wasn't. She was very healthy, but they kept trying to label her 'high risk' even though she'd go back with information proving them wrong. Her doctor would get defensive, then concede that maybe she didn't have that particular condition, but the latest test showed she did have another one that would require further testing. The entire pregnancy was wrought with frustration and far more work than any woman should have to do in pregnancy. These parents were not displeased with their experience. I could conceive of so much better and wanted more for them, but what matters is their perception, not mine. They had their best birth.

Had they listened to this doctor's actions instead of his words, and listened to that small voice inside that cried out after every visit, who knows how much more might they have enjoyed their journey? Ironically, the reasoning behind seeking out this provider and consenting to all of the testing was to get reassurance that everything was 'alright' so they'd feel safe.

If you want a comfortable, empowering, safe and joyous birth, but all of your friends have to tell are horrible stories, pain, and sick babies, don't do what they did! Doing the same thing over-and-over but expecting a different outcome is the definition of insanity! Talk to women who rave about their births, who had alert babies that nursed with no problems, who talk about how wonderful it was, who had smooth postpartum transitions…then find out who their caregiver was!

In smaller towns, it may be easier to discern who the safest providers are. Say in one of our sample counties, there is only one hospital with three obstetricians. If said hospital has a nearly 40% cesarean rate we already know one thing…that at that hospital many more mothers will face a surgical birth than WHO recommends. Surgical births have a greater mortality rate than natural births. Knowing, as we do now, that such high cesarean rates means preventable deaths, we can see that there are many problems with choosing to give birth here.

Inadvertently, this tells us something else. It illustrates the safety of birth and how irrational our fear of birth actually is.

Counties on a Michigan map in 2003 showed that there were 9.8 to 22.2 baby deaths per one thousand births...higher infant death rates than Cuba, Kuwait, Hungary, Bulgaria, Russia and Romania. Simplifying then, in a county with one hospital delivering only one hundred or so babies a year, it could take about 10 years to compile accurate data. On the low end, (9.8/1,000) that would be only one or less baby deaths a year. That doesn't seem like much...unless it's your baby (as caregivers like to point out to justify inappropriate technology).

However, not all doctors practice the same. Many are working diligently to bring their practices in line with evidence-based care recommendations. What if one doctor, in our example, uses a non-invasive approach when possible, utilizing integrative therapies, and has brought her cesarean rate down to 12%?

If this is your doctor, your work is done. Happy birth-day! When this doctor says, "I may not agree with you, but we'll do it your way unless there is a medical indication for intervention." She means it. How do you know? Her numbers don't lie. Her actions back up her words.

If this is not your doctor, you still have gained a lot of insight into the other two doctors. If the above physician has a 12% cesarean rate and the hospital has only two other doctors but a nearly 40% cesarean rate, how high are the rates of the other doctors? So now, you have several options:

Do nothing, keep with your original choice and hope nothing bad happens. This basically means you are playing the odds. Remember: Don't wager more than you can afford to lose. If you had a million dollars, would you bet on 1 in 3 or 50/50 odds that you'd lose? Why do it with your child's life? As with any choice, ask yourself, 'is it in the best interest of the child?' Am I making

90

this choice because it's just easier to do nothing or out of fear? If so, that might be something to explore before the birth.

Stay with this doctor but research every recommendation, fighting for evidence-based care at every visit. Do-able, but exhausting. In a relationship of equals this is more likely to be a workable solution, but doctor-patient relationships are seldom equal. If the relationship is based on a power struggle, someone must lose, usually the least powerful. Wouldn't a win/win, cooperative relationship be more desirable?

Change caregivers. Maybe more than once. Possibly extending out of a convenient geographical area. In a bigger city where a woman is probably a faceless chart this may not be difficult. In a small town, uncomfortable social moments may crop up from such a decision. When the subject is the life of a child vs. saving face, again, the question is, "What is in the best interest of the child?" We pay our caregivers a lot of money to work for us. It is reasonable to expect well-researched care. It is responsible parenting to seek it elsewhere if caregiver is unwilling to provide it. Good doctors have already taken the initiative to keep up on the scientific literature…reward them for their efforts and it's a win/win situation.

Another option is hiring a midwife. Ask the same questions of a midwife that you would of a physician attending your birth. Frequently you won't have to ask. Midwives often provide their statistics at the initial visit without needing to be asked. If the midwife determines at that visit that for some reason you are a poor candidate for a home birth, she may be able to refer you to a sympathetic doctor. Think about what it is you want at a birth.

Find a freestanding birth center. This is a birth center independent from and outside of a hospital. Some consider this a compromise for those that don't want to be at home, but don't want to be in the hospital either. Others choose freestanding birth centers on any of their own plentiful merits. They provide a homey atmosphere within the midwifery model of care, usually with physician backup.

There may come a time when all birth providers share important information voluntarily as providers, proud of their stats, do now. Or, other states may enact laws to protect the consumer, wherein the health department collects the data and provides it to mothers in a brochure so that mothers can make informed decisions as New York has.

No one would dispute that safety is first-and-foremost in choosing a pregnancy care provider, but there are other considerations.

One concern is financial. One questioned often asked at an initial visit with a midwife, or during a phone pre-interview is "Do you take insurance?" Insurance companies that aren't owned and operated by doctors are seeing a financial motive for covering home birth and birth centers, albeit at a snails pace, as more women choose these options.

Parents need to look at the higher short-term cost of inappropriate technology as well as the long-term financial picture use of these technology paints. With a higher number of birth injuries and cesareans in what we think of as 'usual' care, parents may well be paying a co-pay on major abdominal surgery instead of a vaginal birth. Many midwives charge about what parents would end up paying out-of-pocket for their hospital birth insurance co-pay for a vaginal birth. For the uninsured or underinsured, the financial choice is easy...physician at an exorbitant price or midwife at a fraction of the cost. My baby's safety was worth what I'd spend on a vacation or save by not smoking...and then some. I know people whose children are starting school who are still paying on their births!

The other problem is of an emotional/relational nature.

Human nature dictates that if I say, "Wisconsin is a great place to live!" someone will take that to mean that that some place else isn't and reply, "What's wrong with Michigan?"

When we make a choice that might be different from what our peers are doing, it can seem to them as if we are questioning their choices, even though it has nothing to do with them.

When all of my choices were different from that of my mother, her response was to ask questions and often she'd say "If I had known that, I would have done a lot of things different." No guilt required on my part or hers. I was doing the best I could with what I had and so did she.

Very often, objections are simply due to ignorance of why parents are making a particular choice or of the facts pertaining to that choice. Families firmly opposed to home birth often become home birth advocates once they were assured of its safety. Fathers and grandfathers become the biggest advocates, taking great pride in their wife's, or daughter's, empowerment.

Evidence-based care can become the norm. With midwives better utilized the US can move up to one of the top three safest countries in which to give birth. Unfortunately, if you are in your childbearing years now, that is not your reality. In fact, without your help, it won't be the reality of your children either. Here are some concrete things you can do to ensure safer care for you and your baby.

Ask:

Do you utilize prenatal testing only when medically indicated?

Are you supportive of dialog regarding my care?

Do you encourage evidence-based childbirth education?

Is your cesarean rate under 15%?

Is your episiotomy rate under 10%?

Is your induction rate under 10%?

Is your VBAC rate at least 70%?

Do you 'allow' pregnancy to go to 42 weeks if baby and I are healthy?

May I labor without a time limit if both my baby and I are tolerating labor well?

Do you allow vaginal birthing of babies deemed "large" via ultrasound?

Do you discourage routine circumcision?

Do you support breastfeeding by not giving out formula samples?

Will you support requests that are not standard protocol, as long as they are reasonable and not medically contraindicated?

Will you allow me to digitally record my birth?

Can I be sure that you will be attending my birth?

If not, would the attending provider share your philosophies?

If your provider responded 'yes' to all 15 questions, you have found a responsible, safe and respectful caregiver. Your own best birth can be expected.

If your provider responded 'yes' to at least 10 of the above question, your caregiver might be willing to work with you, but a pathological view of birth may be unconsciously be under that willingness. Clear communication and a little more work on your part may be required for an optimal experience. Give them a month or two. If, after attempts at being a partner in your care, you are not being met halfway, find someone who is willing to meet you there.

If your provider responded 'yes' to 5 or less, 6 or 7 months is simply not enough time to bring this caregiver around. Remaining with this caregiver means there is a high probability you will be a statistic in the sad state of American maternity care. The chance that you will have a safe, dignified and empowering birth is next to nil.

Also, keep in mind that underreporting, not just of mortality and morbidity rates, but of certain procedures, is the norm in our health care system, as evidenced by a quick web search of the word 'underreporting'. Verify 'internal sources' with independent sources of information. There are often huge discrepancies between the two statistics.

Finally, remember to be sure words and actions say the same thing.

"IN OUR EVERY DELIBERATION, WE MUST CONSIDER THE IMPACT OF OUR DECISIONS ON THE NEXT SEVEN GENERATIONS."
FROM: THE GREAT LAW OF THE IROQUOIS CONFEDERACY

Journal Exploration:

List 3 behaviors that intellectually you know are not beneficial to your baby or yourself, but you continue to do anyway. Determine why it's detrimental to an optimal birth outcome, then identify what unconscious motivators may be fueling the behavior.

Behavior#1: _____

Unconscious motivator:

_____

Behavior #2:

_____

Unconscious motivator:

_____

Behavior #3:

_____

Unconscious motivator:

_____

PART TWO

Motivation

OUR ACTIONS ARE BASED ON WHAT WE THINK WE KNOW
ABOUT BIRTH. NOW THAT YOU HAVE AN IDEA OF WHAT
MAKES BIRTH SAFER, DO YOU KNOW HOW TO MAKE IT
HAPPEN FOR YOU? DO YOU KNOW HOW TO BE MORE
COMFORTABLE? ARE YOU READY TO EXPLORE YOUR
OPTIONS? PART TWO BUILDS MOMENTUM IN YOUR
NEWFOUND MOTIVATION.

CHAPTER 4

(pre) Creation

How can America be one of the most technologically advanced countries on Earth and *not* be one of the safest places to give birth? One reason may be simple American hubris that we are known for throughout the world. Another reason may be that our technological capability has surpassed our ethics or common sense.

In any case, how is it that American parents can be under the assumption that they are safer due to the technology, when all of the evidence says otherwise? The technology has the potential to save lives. It seems to make sense that better technology means better outcomes. So why isn't the case?

Accountability is paramount to the solution. Everyone who shapes the current system of maternity care, from the doctors, to the nurses, to midwives, to the consumer, needs to be accountable for their part in the reality we have.

This is not about blame. Blame is part of the problem. Blame and accountability are not the same. Blame releases us from accountability because it puts responsibility for outcomes outside of ourselves. If we can tell ourselves we had no hand in breaking it, we don't have to fix it. "I'm only doing what the women demand" is blame. "My doctor didn't tell me" is blame. "I'm only doing my job" is blame.

However, we are all responsible. Without acknowledging that our choices matter, we won't make better choices.

This means good, bad, fair or unfair, every choice you make as a parent affects the outcome of your birth; likewise for caregivers.

There are no inconsequential actions. If you've never considered this before, it's essential that it is understood now, because now you are making choices for two.

It's important to understand that this applies to normal, healthy women. No one is suggesting that illness or injury is within your control—though there are a number of situations in which it might be prevented.

What is true is that we construct our own reality with every choice we make...or don't make. By the end of this chapter you will understand what you control, and what you only control your reaction to. If you are thinking to yourself right now that there is no way your feelings of fear, your lack of confidence or some pregnancy 'condition' you've been diagnosed with is under your control, keep reading. You will be surprised to learn how much really is. I promise.

However, you have to consider there may be a grain of truth to the idea that birth can be safe and comfortable or you'll be giving your power away. Don't victimize yourself by accepting the illusion that birth is always a dangerous medical event that can only be handled by pros. Barring unforeseen circumstances, no one can control your birth process unless you allow it.

If you really want a healthy pregnancy and joyful birth, and you truly understand that you are the one in control, then you must examine what you have or haven't done so far to create the outcome you want.

How do you know where your current choices will lead if you are newly pregnant for the first time? Do you have the same attitudes and hold the same opinions as your friends? Most of us do. What were their outcomes? I'm not talking about a healthy baby. That should be the expectation of most parents. Nature is very efficient at the survival game. There are very few things that actually go wrong in pregnancy.

100

There are many things that could…but not that many that actually do very often in a well-nourished healthy baby-momma.

Past behavior is the best indicator of future outcomes. So, the choices of people you know have usually resulted in healthy babies. That's the good news. What did it cost them? Not 'what did it cost' in literally dollars, though the cost of conventional maternity care is a disgrace. Midwives deliver the same results or better for far less. But what did it cost them personally? Did they have postpartum depression? Did they have trouble bonding or nursing? Is the baby healthy or been plagued with ear infections, digestive problems, behavioral problems? Does the mother have an episiotomy scar that is affecting daily living? Did she have to try to mother a newborn and heal from major abdominal surgery at the same time? Did she 'almost die' having her baby? Did she need to be 'rescued?' While there are certainly circumstances where bad things really do happen and those types of statements might be true, it is also true that oftentimes circumstances were created that didn't have to be. These are called 'iotrogenic' (doctor caused) or 'nosocomial' (hospital caused). Facing these situations in what should have been an uncomplicated birth is a high price tag for the normal birth that is a woman's right.

When we stop seeing these as created difficulties, we begin to see them as 'normal.' We say, 'That's the price you pay for a healthy baby.' Many of the problems mothers face during hospital birth happen infrequently in the midwifery model, but the woman still gets the baby 'prize' and so much more out of their mothering experience. How fair is that? Why aren't women mad that they have to 'pay' for something that is already theirs?

Obstetricians indulge in a little self-reflection as well to understand why they are the most sued profession. By taking some responsibility for it instead of blaming lawyers and patients, they can address the real issues and become part of the solution.

We don't live in a culture that supports the idea that we are responsible for the outcomes of our actions. Not accepting responsibility means we can't learn and grow. It means we must entertain new ideas about victimization. Anita's story is a prime example.

Anita was a smart, strong woman. She took an independent childbirth class and read books about making her experience better. She decided she didn't want to make a big fuss about the all the prenatal testing. It was easier just to do what her doctor said. She knew she could choose a midwife, and said she wanted to, but her husband wouldn't 'allow' it. Besides, she was healthy and took great care of herself. The tests wouldn't show anything bad.

Her triple screen test indicated that her baby had a chromosomal abnormality. The recommendation was to do further testing. She read up on further testing, only to discover there was an unacceptably high chance, to her, of her losing the baby due to the test. The next test was also no more reliable than the first, although she did agree to an extra ultrasound, which confirmed the diagnoses. There was nothing to be done about the problem. She was advised to abort.

She couldn't bring herself to do that. She was under an incredible amount of stress, was constantly being told that now she was high risk and would need a cesarean, though a cesarean would not change the outcome for either her or the child. She got genetic counseling. She took classes on caring for a special needs child. She was fearful about whether or not she could love enough and how all of this would affect the rest of her life.

What a relief when her baby boy was born completely healthy, right? Of course, that's all that matters. Except that the pointless assault on her emotional and psychological health, or the toll this took on her life, negatively impacted her work and her family significantly. Her marriage didn't survive the stress. Maybe the marriage would have dissolved somewhere down the road anyway.

Maybe not.

You can believe that what's wrong with the system has nothing to do with you. That woman was not the first who went through this with this particular doctor and she wasn't the last. She asked questions, but she didn't act on the answers. She sacrificed so much of what should have been the happiest time of her life with unnecessary stress. Were there long term repercussions with bonding? Did the stress hormones produced by her body negatively affect her baby's brain development as doctors and scientists postulate? (Wirth, 2001) What would be the point in knowing for sure? What's done is done. Unless other parents would be spared her torment, why go there? Would your decisions be affected if you knew for sure her child had suffered the consequence of this situation? Would you think it couldn't happen to you? She knew the reputation of this doctor and that's exactly what she thought.

Parents can keep feeling as if they are mistreated and powerless and they will be mistreated and powerless. They can shut their eyes to books full of scientific studies about our current birth technology and the evidence of misuse contaminating the process of birth. They can insist that anyone who would question the status quo is just wrong.

What if they aren't? If the 'normal' choices are right, and the 'weird' choices are wrong, why are the ones making the 'wrong' choices having the faster, more comfortable births and sometimes even a blissful experience of motherhood?

You can be angry that it seems unfair that so few women have 'fairy tale' births, or you can become Cinderella. You have to be willing to be flexible in your position and willing to admit maybe there are other possibilities.

You can keep doing what you are doing, what all of your cesarean friends have done, if you want a surgical birth...preparing to deal with all of the difficulties that it entails.

OR you can decide that there might be an alternative for you.

Let others blame the system, the books they read or the bodies they have been led to believe are deficient or defective. Be the one to truly change your life. Stand up and take what's yours. Do it for your baby. Stop looking in the wrong place for answers only you have.

Realize from this moment on that every decision you make from this point on has consequences to your birth. Also realize you had this power from the beginning of your pregnancy, as well. As you consider that past choices led to present results, you may have to adjust personal perceptions. It's important that you remember 'responsibility' is not the same as 'fault'. Allow yourself the space to acknowledge how your actions affect your present circumstance, then release the negativity that affects your life. Let your 'self talk' be different. Remind yourself that you were designed to birth with daily affirmations such as:

My body knows how to build and birth this baby just as it knows how to do other natural and normal things like breathe and sleep.

I trust my body to communicate my birthing needs just as it tells me when I need food by communicating through hunger.

I have already been entrusted with the growth and well-being of this baby...I am strong and capable enough to consciously join in choices to that end.

Birth beliefs, thoughts, choices, and unhealthy behaviors become yours to change if you can recognize how you may have been complicit in your mistreatment simply because you didn't know you had options. You have the ability to purposefully change the birth experience you create.

Resolve to analyze the events of your pregnancy as they relate to the choices you make. Sometimes they won't align (sometime stuff just happens), but you'll be surprised how often they do.

104

Doing so reframes how you interact with your partner, your caregiver and other mothers. "Why me?" becomes "Why not?" You will begin to wonder, "How can I change this situation or my reaction to it?" "What are my options and do I have all of the information I need to explore each one?" If you don't know your options, you don't have any.

If you've been focusing on what you don't want, it should become clear that you can also plan for success. Success is what you want it to be. It isn't about what anybody else thinks or what is 'right' or 'wrong'. How you feel when all is said and done reflects if the choice was right for you. Do you feel confident, strong, and competent? These are indications you have made the right choice for yourself, your baby and your situation. Or do you feel uncertain and vulnerable to feelings of guilt? This may indicate you've made decisions that you knew or suspected to be right for someone else but perhaps not you.

It's certainly easier to place blame than to be accountable. Our culture supports the victim mentality. That's why malpractice rates are so high and frivolous lawsuits are out of control. By not accepting responsibility for how we are affected by our own actions, we don't have to expect more of ourselves.

It would be easy to believe that we are victims of the broken obstetrical system because of the obstetricians, but that's not entirely true. The specialty of obstetrics developed because sometimes we need them. We must accept that often, inappropriate technology is used because we ask for it.

Doctors must take responsibility for allowing parents to dictate inappropriate care, for sure. However, the hypocrisy of saying that the epidural or cesarean rates are only so high because women demand it, yet meeting reasonable requests with snide remarks like, 'where did you go to medical school?' (as has happened to so many women) has to stop. Would an internal surgeon open you up and look around just because you demanded exploratory surgery?

The system is partially shaped by the women in it, partly by caregivers. At least two other forces are also a factor… economics and fear.

Economics and Fear

Inappropriate technology used in the name of defensive medicine exists because parents sue doctors. Not just doctors with bad judgment or malicious intent, but good ones too. All doctors (and parents!) are being punished in this complex situation.

It may seem that the system is unfair, that you were only doing what you were told; that just because birth in the should as safe and satisfying experience in hospital as it is in birthing centers and at home, it is. Without acting toward what you want though, it's unlikely to happen. The odds are just against it right now, which means you must actively work toward the outcome of a healthy, whole child and an unwounded body and soul for yourself at the end of your journey.

If you don't want to hear that, you aren't alone. Ask your sisters and friends about their births. They may have a gorgeous, healthy baby…but what unnecessary sacrifices were they asked to make? Did they sacrifice their dignity? Integrity? Their sex life? Their marriage? Further childbearing capability? Their child's learning potential? What justifications do they use to make it okay? Is blame involved, including blaming of themselves? Many women internalize blame, and I'm afraid there are many ways that this is encouraged in the current system. It deflects blame that could cost someone cold, hard cash. Accountability is essential; blame is not acceptable.

Sacrifice is a part of motherhood so we accept it without question. Certain sacrifices are a mother's lot in life: sleep deprivation, a change in body structure resulting from growing an entire human being within your body and birthing it into the world. However, far too many women are being required to sacrifice far too much far too often. It's up to you to determine how much unwarranted sacrifice you are willing to heap on top of what is already inherent in motherhood. To bear more than your fair share, assuming the role of victim by your own free will starts you out on your new path with a deficit that makes the job so much harder.

It's self-preservation to try to escape accountability, to justify and rationalize poor treatment. We have a hard time being objective during pregnancy when we are so emotionally involved, and often have unconscious fear of the unknown guiding our decisions. However, we cannot face challenges and come up with solutions hindered by a lack of objectivity. It's imperative to adopt new ways of thinking.

You can't solve a problem with blame. You can't just coast along because the truth doesn't fit with the current prevailing birth beliefs. Doing nothing is doing something. If you are feeling frightened, confused, overwhelmed, unsure or powerless about how your pregnancy is progressing, how your birth will end up or what to expect from your new life with baby, you need to accept that you have the power to change so much of it!

You choose the food that builds your baby.
You the books you read, if any.
You control which images of birth you accept as reality.
You choose what kind of childbirth class you take, if any.
You choose your care provider.
You choose how you will allow your caregiver to treat you.
You choose what tests you will allow.
You determine the level of understanding you have of your care.
You choose your birth location.
You choose to smoke, take drugs or drink alcohol…or not.
You choose natural birth, or not.

Can you add to this list?

Remember, blame and responsibility are not the same. Disregarding the consequences of decisions, or intentionally inflicting harm knowingly by taking action known to be potentially harmful, may warrant blame. Responsibility means being accountable for actions that were under your control. Intent makes the difference.

Guilt is often the end-result of blame-worthy behavior. Guilt is a message from our inner self that says we knew we did something wrong. It is meant to help us navigate difficult situations so that even if we make mistakes, we learn from them and don't repeat them.

As seen in previous chapters, there is a need to be willing to look closely at feelings of guilt because, unfortunately, misplaced guilt is common. Neither real guilt nor misplaced guilt is meant to be a carried for a lifetime. The purpose of true guilt is to alter behavior. Once we recognize it, we decide to do better next time, we let it go and we move on. Misplaced guilt simply has no purpose.

This should be liberating news. If you really don't have control in pregnancy, birth, or breastfeeding experience you can release feelings of guilt that were not yours to carry. If you made a bad choice knowing there was a better one, you can allow the guilt to guide you in the future to make the better choice, and release the guilt that's done its job.
You can't change the past, you can only choose your reaction to it and learn from it. Letting regret or misplaced guilt impact future decisions only hurts you. It's far better to be pro-active in making sound decisions you know you'll feel strong about, no matter what the outcome.

Has your caregiver belittled or berated you for asking intelligent questions? Have you avoided asking questions because you feared he or she would? Were you coerced into dropping a great childbirth class because your provider played a power trip and said you couldn't continue with his or her practice if you didn't? Only you have the power to change your the direction of your care.

The good news is, you have the power.

Here's an illustration of just how thoughts and feelings affect your birth.

The mind affects the body in very concrete, biological ways. In this instance, we are talking about the body that your child calls 'home.'

Do you blush easily? If so, it is a thought that causes the physiological response of blood to rushing to your face. Do you get an upset stomach from stress? Your thoughts are triggering a physical response in your body and you make more stomach acid.

It's more important to understand the mind/body connection in pregnancy and birth than any other time. It can make the difference between painless, drug-free birthing and suffering.

Your choices now literally program your experience later. Please do the work you need to do to get the result you want. Getting a handle on any negative 'self talk' now will make parenting easier and more enjoyable later.

Taking your reclaimed power takes practice. It's easy to get overly excited about empowerment, to start demanding better treatment. It's important to find the balance that culminates in building respectful relationships with care providers...not alienation.

Consider that 'what comes around goes around.' How you approach your caregiver means a lot. It's all right to give people the benefit of the doubt.

Do you want to be a partner in your care? Mutual respect is the foundation.

What is your communication style? What is your partner's? What is your care provider's?

Nice:

This is the 'dream' caregiver. Doctor or midwife, this care provider is the perfect fit. They seem to like everyone. They are open to new ideas and treat everyone as valuable. Even if they disagree with you, they'll tell you they disagree, respecting that this is your birth and your life. If there is a medical reason for something, they will explain everything to your satisfaction. The important thing here is they back it up. Others may say it, but words and deeds contradict each other. Not here. This is someone who will go the extra mile to look up new information so they can give you a fresh perspective, even changing their thoughts on something if the evidence supports it. They actually respect a parent who does their homework. Parents who communicate in this style are respectful and inquisitive. They want to know why tests are suggested and want to research the applicability of each intervention independently before discussing their options with their care provider and making a decision.

Not so nice:

These people take everything personally and become defensive and/or offended easily. Asking a simple question may bring on a condescending and hostile attitude. Manipulative tactics will be used to get you to comply. This person doesn't expect you to question anything and will personally attack if you do, often with 'If you want to kill your baby...' sort of maneuvers.

As clients, these people don't ask questions, they make accusations.

Arrogant:

These people hate being wrong. They don't get angry about questions though, because they deftly avoid them, not really taking you seriously. You may not realize your questions have not been answered until you're on the way home. If you persist, the response is likely to be "Where did you go to medical school?" (Though these are the people who also say they only use unnecessary technology because the patient demands it!)

110

When this type of communicator is a client, it is a nightmare for the care provider. These people refuse reasonable recommendations and ignore efforts to explain why or why not a particular intervention may be justified.

Clueless:
As caregivers, these people are just plain inattentive. They seem distracted because they are, and usually what's on their mind has nothing to do with you. When presented with a birth plan they'll say "Sure, sure, anything you want". Don't expect it though…he or she hasn't even actually looked at it and won't 'find time' before your birth.

In mothers, these would be the ones for whom the realization that there's a baby in there doesn't hit until the baby is in their arms. These mothers often have difficult births because they don't prepare at all…they just assume someone else always takes care of stuff. Fear takes over in the end when reality sets in.

Controlling:
These domineering people are insufferable because they don't just know everything, they presume to know how you should think and what you should feel. They tell you, too. These doctors will 'fire' you as a patient if so much as look at an unauthorized book or set foot in a class of which they don't control the content. Loss of control over you is not tolerated.

Women who are perfectionists of this sort may have difficult births if they can't lighten up. Motherhood is all about adaptability and if that realization isn't made, these mothers are miserable.

High Drama:
In care providers, this means nothing is ever simple. A stitch in your side requires a battery of tests. Requesting any deviation of the usual routine is likely to be met with "I don't like to deliver dead babies!" There is a catastrophe around every corner and he or she is the only thing keeping you safe. Don't expect evidence-based care from this

provider...he or she doesn't look at scientific evidence, but acts on adrenaline and fear.

Parents that fall into this category wear their caregivers out! They think they have every complication or illness they've ever read about and call their care provider constantly with new complaints.

Victim:
If this person is a care provider, nothing is their fault. Routine technology harmful? They only do it because patients make them! The lawyers are out to get them, the patients are out to get them, you make them do it! Everyone's out to get them anyway, what difference would competency make? They won't bother to look at new information because as far as they are concerned, they're damned if they do and damned if they don't.

Mothers who identify with this way of engaging are likely to just go along with everything, asking no questions, thinking everything bad in life always happens to them and there is nothing they can do to change it. These parents may seem like a caregiver's dream...as long as everything goes as planned. If the parent inadvertently later gains knowledge about evidence-based care, parents in the group are the 'why me-s' and blamers...they are the ones who most often sue.

Analysts:
These people are scientists at heart. They love knowledge and they have excellent critical thinking skills. Care providers in this group love it when you bring them new information that can be substantiated and incorporate it into their practice.

These types are also dream clients when the caregiver is practicing evidence-based care. They look up what you tell them to verify it themselves but each time they get confirmation they trust more, the relationship strengthened. These clients rarely sue because they feel that everyone played fair and know that sometimes, bad things still happen, though the odds are in their favor with knowledge.

Care providers not practicing evidence-based care hate these patients because it makes them work too hard.

We all have all of these traits and many more besides. In balance, they make up a positive interaction. Out of balance, they can affect your decisions in ways you might not want.

Choosing to remain in an unhealthy relationship with a caregiver is as harmful as remaining in an unhealthy relationship with anyone else. Make no mistake; even choosing not to act in a bad situation is a choice. Each prenatal choice leads to the one-and-only entry into the world your child will make. Be consciously aware of what you are creating.

It's natural to resist change. At one point in our ancestral history, survival was contingent on the known and familiar. Our brains work the same way now. It would be completely normal to feel discomfort as new ideas urge you to change how you think and behave. Other people may even react to you differently as you begin acting more confidently. It will start to feel more natural as you get more used to it!

By being willing to embrace, or at least explore, new thought, you will be amazed at how much you enjoy your pregnancy, and eventually, your birth; after that new motherhood. Being judgmental or dismissive just because ideas are new or unusual will deprive you of nature's gifts to new mothers.

Chloe's story is one of this reclamation of power.

Chloe was a strong young woman. She and her husband read everything they could about birth early in their pregnancy. In their second trimester, they decided to see a midwife.

In their community, the medical establishment refused to provide back up to qualified midwives. This put the couple in the undesirable position of continuing prenatal care with their doctor without informing him of their home birth plans in order to be able to transfer to the hospital in the event of an emergency. The midwife would have preferred a better arrangement as well, but it was better than the alternative of no emergency plan at all, so she went along with the decision.

One day, Chloe appeared at her midwife's door, days before her next scheduled prenatal/midwifery appointment, miserable and scared. During a routine doctor's visit, she had been told she was in premature labor. This diagnosis was made on the basis of a (useless, routine) (Weiss, 2010) vaginal exam that her doctor told her showed dilation of two-three cm (not necessarily unusual at 36 weeks), as well as an electronic-fetal monitor strip (also proven to be useless in improving outcomes without medical indication) (Alfirevic, Devane, Gyte, 2007) that showed she was having contractions (which she didn't feel—had never felt). From that visit (where she was told all sorts of horrifying stories of the effects of pre-maturity) she was sent to the hospital. There she was given IV terbutaline to stop premature labor (which has been proven ineffective in stopping true premature labor, as well as too risky) (Wildner, 2002; FDA, 2011) and then sent home with an oral medication, Brethine (which the Physician's Desk Reference says not to use in pregnancy). After only a few days on the drug, this mother, who had taken excellent care of herself and been healthy up until that last visit, began to feel very ill. Her heart raced, her baby moved non-stop as its heart rate did the same. Nausea kept her from eating and drinking. She couldn't sleep.

Her midwife sadly informed her that once drugs were introduced, this became a medical event. Midwives deal with normal pregnancy and birth, which this no longer was. The midwife offered to accompany Chloe to the hospital as labor support for the birth, but could not help her at home while she was on the medication. Besides, Chloe had not reached 37 weeks, which is the earliest midwives will allow home birth.

At that point, Chloe confessed to having reduced the dosage of the drug of her own volition. She asked if the midwife would attend her at home if there was time to clear the drug from her system and if she could make it past the 37 week mark. Her midwife conferred with her partner and agreed, if those conditions were met, and there were no complications resulting from the treatment, they could do it at home. All of this was contingent on whether the mother really was in premature labor. After checking Chloe's cervix and finding it high and closed, the midwife determined that Chloe had never been in premature labor.

Chloe called her midwife a few days later. Protein was present on her urine dipstick, her blood pressure was up and swelling had worsened. These are all of the symptoms of pre-eclampsia, which is very dangerous. They are also signs of a compromised liver (one of the risks of terbutaline, according to the Physician's Desk Reference).

Chloe had reached 37 weeks, but she would still have to birth in the hospital.

At the hospital, the doctor was rude, rough and disrespectful. He didn't ask Chloe or her husband how they might like to proceed or offer any options, which they knew were available from their reading.

He told them what he would do, then abruptly left, leaving orders with the nurse to break Chloe's water and start pitocin.

Chloe asked her midwife if she could help her use hypnosis to bring her blood pressure down long enough to go to a different hospital. She knew that allowing the interventions this doctor was intent on using would, in all likelihood, result in a cesarean. After discussion with the understanding that a cesarean might still be an option as sick as she now was, it was agreed to at least try.

Relaxation brought her blood pressure down to normal levels. Chloe got dressed and was ready to sign out AMA (against medical advice) when her doctor returned. He was furious. He yelled at her. He accused her of trying to kill her baby. He detailed all of the tragedies that would befall her if she walked out the door. He not only made her sign the AMA form, but he made her write out and sign a letter he dictated, stating that she knew she was killing her baby by making this choice. This brave mother stayed relaxed throughout his entire tirade and walk out.

She went to a different hospital. She explained what had happened, all the while, remaining calm and keeping her blood pressure down.

Once settled into the new hospital, Chloe did have medication to keep her blood pressure down, and she did have low dose pitocin to get labor started. It took a long time to get labor going…she was only 37 weeks and had never really been in premature labor…but eventually her own body took over. She had to work hard to stay relaxed as her condition made it impossible to move to a more comfortable position and she needed to be hooked up to two IVs for true medical indications.

But she did it. She had her own best birth. It didn't turn out as she planned, but she knew that she made the best choices for her baby and avoided what would have been an unnecessary surgery.

Journal Exploration:

Write a letter to your baby. Explain why you are making choices you are making. Do you find any excuses in what you might say? Are there really options you just aren't willing to look at for one reason or another? What reasons to you give to justify the sacrifices your baby might be asked to make for your decisions? Ask your baby if these are the choices he/she would make if he/she could. Go into the still, wise self with three deep breaths to release tension, then writing with your non-dominant hand (to access the subconscious mind more easily), explore these same questions from your baby's perspective.

CHAPTER 5

Human Nature

In previous chapters, we've looked at the safety of birth in America. We've examined the role fear plays in our decision making process, as parents and professionals alike. We've seen how skillfully our subconscious beliefs manipulate our actions. We now clearly recognize how belief affects perception, which is reality.

It's a lot to absorb. You may be noticing you view the world a little differently now that you've done the work in the first chapters.

You may have changed some behaviors. You may have revised some long held beliefs and are wondering why others do what they do. You may be thinking differently, but have not put the new knowledge to work, and wonder at your own reluctance to make changes.

Why do parents support a system that in large measure treats them poorly and puts their children at risk? Why do doctors perpetuate a system that continues to generate more lawsuits than any other profession? Why do media producers and editors perpetuate the fear by portraying birth in frightening ways? Why do midwives keep trying to improve a system that doesn't seem to want to improve when the effort might land them in jail? Why do lawyers prosecute the midwives when every shred of credible scientific evidence supports midwifery for healthy mothers and babies?

All of us play a part in the system we now have to deal with. The blame cannot be placed with just one group. Responsibility must be met by all, and all must hold the others accountable for their portion of the problem if we are ever to find a solution. We must step up to the plate for our mothers and babies.

We all do what we do for the same reason. On some level there is a perceived reward for our behavior. Sometimes it's obvious, sometimes not.

Our behavior creates our outcomes. Success is measured by results. Is what we are doing, and have been doing, making birth safer? Is what we're doing helping produce happy, healthy, well adjusted children? Is what we're doing helping doctors care for high-risk patients and midwives care for healthy mothers? If our results are indicative, no, what we're doing certainly isn't working!

Mothers are so afraid of a natural, gloriously designed process that they are choosing to not feel a thing, detaching emotionally and physically from the most rewarding effort they'll ever make in their lives.

It doesn't look like it's working—so why do we keep doing the same things over-and-over again? Why are we not learning from our mistakes? Why do our collective behaviors create results benefiting so few? Denial is certainly part of the problem.

And here is one example of how this is perpetuated.

A popular morning news program ran a series called "Having a Baby Today" in April of 2003. In one portion of this series a physician was interviewed and several opinions were expressed. These opinions were based on faulty core assumptions and contradicted by the scientific literature. When I told a friend that I was going to write to the show and point out these inaccuracies, I was asked, "If what she said wasn't factual, how could she say it?" I asked my friend, "Did you question her advice?" The response was "No." The show didn't verify the facts, why would the viewers?

If you had seen it, would you have questioned the advice? Probably not. Most wouldn't. After all, she's a doctor, on the show to help us make safe decisions, right?

Her assertion home birth isn't safe for healthy mothers and babies is patently and demonstrably false. Her assertion that elective cesareans are a good thing because they save pelvic floor function is also not supported according to US researchers reporting in Obstetrics and Gynecology (Buchsbaum, et al, 2002), which states that women who have never experienced childbirth are just as likely as those who have given birth to develop urinary incontinence, a finding that casts doubts on the theory that vaginal deliveries increase the risk of incontinence. What does cause pelvic floor damage is episiotomy, still routine for many doctors.

This sort of thing happens all over the nation every day. Blindly accepting opinion as fact keeps the erroneous beliefs in play. Few have been willing to admit the existing dysfunction. Yet, make no mistake…no matter how logical or rational you may be, if you aren't part of the solution, you are part of the problem.

We know that in pregnancy, diet and exercise are two of the most important factors in outcome. What are you growing your baby on? Are you growing your baby on whole, fresh foods, or junk?

We know that smoking is responsible for numerous, potentially fatal, pregnancy complications and childhood illnesses. Have you stopped? Have you eliminated as much second-hand smoke from your home and work environments as possible?

We know stress is at least partially responsible for several pregnancy complications. What are you doing to create a peaceful environment for you and your baby?

We know the elements of safe childbearing are:

1. Good nutrition
2. Skillful Midwifery
3. Home birth with skilled midwives
4. Natural Childbirth
5. Breastfeeding (Stewart, 1981)

What kind of commitment have you made to your baby's safety based on this knowledge? Are your choices based on scientific evidence or obstetric myths?

To create your own best birth, you need to stop behaving in ways that interfere with what you want, and begin behaving in ways that advance you toward the better birth you desire.

How do you know what you are doing is working for you? Ask yourself: Are you fearful and anxious? If you think you're not, allow yourself a little honesty about what drives your decisions. A 'just in case' philosophy is built on fear. Testing for conditions that you are not at risk for, and have no symptoms of, is fear-based. Prenatal visits that focus on things that might go wrong instead of what is right are fear-based.

Prenatal visits that leave you crying or with a wiggly feeling in your belly mean your intuition is screaming at you!

Logically, we know this isn't what we want, but we feel powerless to change. Parents do what they do out of love, first-and-foremost, and safety. But if that is true, as we know it is, why make decisions that are proven unsafe? It seems illogical.

We come back to fear and belief. They believe that they are making the safest choices, yet fear is the root of their choice.

This may not be a conscious fear. Though many will come to a childbirth class fully willing to admit that they are (consciously) terrified, I believe in most mothers the fear is subconsciously lurking. Only about one quarter of the mothers giving birth annually even come to classes. There are a number of reasons for this, but if you ask a first-time mother who has the means, transportation and support why she didn't attend, she'd probably tell you she doesn't see a reason. Either she believes what will be, will be, because she has no control anyway, or she will say that she just expects everything to be fine because pregnancy and birth are normal and she is healthy…yet she makes choices that contradicts this because they are based in a 'just in case' mentality, or perhaps she just believes someone else (her doctor) can provide a perfect outcome regardless of whether she contributes or contaminates the process. Healthy mothers who get mad at anyone who suggests that fear is part of their process, all the while seeing a surgeon for a natural function, are contradicting themselves.

It's all right to admit to being afraid. We all fear the unknown. To what degree we allow it to impact decisions is what's important. It's whether we let the fear make our choices, or be the impetus to seek other options so that the fear doesn't surface later to cause problems.

Those that start out consciously acknowledging fear at least can deal with preemptively. Denial of fear allows it to sit in waiting. The current system provides ample opportunity for this to become a problem, even if it has been kept at bay for most of the pregnancy. The last few weeks of pregnancy, and labor itself, are when the majority of women will face their unconscious fears, because that is when inappropriate birth technology is abused the most. By that time, how many women are willing, or able, to question their 'low tech if you want me to be' caregiver who suddenly seems to have a personality transplant? The confidence the parents thought they had disappears in an instant. The 'just in case' (fear-based) philosophy they convinced themselves had nothing to do with fear is suddenly 'proved' to be necessary because some test led to some other test that led to some intervention that led to a very real (and created, not encountered) complication. They haven't prepared themselves on how to maneuver this kind of scenario…it wasn't going to happen to them. Since it did happen, they convince themselves they are part of that small percentage of people for whom the technology is essential.

The way that this 'of course pregnancy is a natural thing, but anything can go wrong at any moment' set up plays out, has been likened to the 'frog in a pot' analogy: A frog tossed into in a pot of boiling water will jump out.

A frog put in a pot of room temperature water with the heat very gradually turned up won't even notice the water getting warm until it's too late to jump.

An independent childbirth educator has seen a lot of frogs. She is probably able to see 'the big picture.' She may have had contact with hundreds of women in your community and may be able to tell you if the local induction rate your OB insists is 'low' is actually 60 or 70% instead of the 10% the World Health Organization suggests. She believes in the normalcy of birth. An independent childbirth class can go a long way toward opening your eyes to the pot of water you may not even know you are in.

Parental birth belief has been explored, but how is it a reward? If we act in ways that support our beliefs, no matter how erroneous they may be, we get what we expect. Having expectations met, even if they are negative consequences, is for some people, better than the unknown. Being fearful does not seem to be a reward, except that fearing what we 'know' seems less scary than the unknown.

Our erroneous beliefs about pregnancy and birth are not the only beliefs in play. Beliefs about authority, about self-esteem and even spiritual beliefs have some affect on how we birth. Do you believe that birth is a natural, biological process? Do you believe current birth technology makes birth safer? Safer than what? Than what it used to be before improvements in sanitation, infection control, nutrition and birth control? Do you know what made (or makes) birth dangerous? Do you believe birth must be painful? Excruciatingly so or manageably? Do you believe if some women have painless birth maybe many, even most, can? Do you believe that the US is one of the safest places in the world to give birth? Does your religion tell you women must suffer to bring forth life? Investigate your beliefs. See if they hold up to the facts. Don't just seek out information that bolsters what you already believe (this is called 'confirmation bias)...see if other views are valid. Some of these we've already discussed in previous chapters, but did you verify them for yourself? Did you dismiss them or simply accept them with no proof? Beliefs are tenacious. If you want to change your experience, you must test your ideas constantly as they reassert themselves in the face of factual information. If they don't hold up to fact, discard them.

What about pain and birth? What would it take to convince you painless, or at least comfortable birth, is possible without drugs? Do you believe women must suffer in birth? 'Suffering' is a judgment of a perception that you can choose to accept or reject. Even if pain is present, one woman may see it as a challenge, while the same level of discomfort may be insufferable for someone who chooses to frame it differently.

An entire chapter is devoted to helping you work on your idea of the perception of pain, so we won't dwell on that here. Just ask yourself, 'Does fear of pain contribute to the choices I am making regarding pregnancy and birth?' The reward there would be freedom from pain, of course, but what if intolerably painful birth is created or rarely encountered, not inherent in the experience?

One reward of abdicating responsibility for that which we are solely responsible for is that it allows us to place blame elsewhere if something goes wrong. This one is a tough one to accept, but the sky rocketing malpractice rate attests to it's validity.

Why would we choose to play the victim? Because we can.

Journal Exploration

It's time to take the opportunity to express possibly unexpressed fears and feelings. Write down what would be left unsaid to each of the following people if you were to die tomorrow: your mother, your father, your partner, your baby, older children (if applicable).

Would you have regrets regarding your pregnancy, birth or parenting?

What are you grateful for?

What might you do differently and how would that impact those above?

Would these be the same things you'd say in 5 years? 10 years? 20 years? Look ahead to your old age. If there is something you feel now that you might regret later, do something about it now. Remember that regret and guilt stem from things we wanted to do but didn't. This is NOT about 'couldn't' situations. If you wanted to do something but circumstances were out of your control, that's entirely different.

Having identified where you might feel regret about your parenting choices, make a list. For each concern, list a least a couple of actions you can take now that will ensure you never have to feel guilt for not doing what your heart and mother's intuition are trying to guide you to do.

Finally, according to Maslow's Hierarchy of Needs, one of our biggest fears is of being excluded. Most people will do almost anything to 'fit in.' Doing what everyone else does, even if we have reservations, seems to be part of our wiring. Social psychologist Stanley Milgram conducted controversial 'obedience experiments' at Yale University in 1961, expecting to show that American subjects would not follow orders that seemed to hurt another person. These experiments showed that indeed good people would do things under orders that they wouldn't do on their own. It seems we humans have sort of a 'pack' mentality. Sports frenzy resulting in riots is an extreme example of this gone awry. Unfortunately, when it comes to making safety decisions for precious babies, we can't afford to be blind followers.

Doctors and Nurses

Everyday, more doctors and nurses question where inappropriate technology has led us. Obviously, they are the minority or conditions would be improving, so what motivates the vast majority of those within the current system? Where are common sense and critical thinking skills?

Just as with parents, it comes back to fear and faulty beliefs. They spend a great deal of time learning about pathology and very little about normal, natural birth. They then see what they expect to see.

They create the reality they perceive to be reality. The medical model sees birth as a disaster waiting to happen, so it's based on fear. Facts that might contradict that belief are dismissed, unless the doctor or nurse is a scientist or non-conformist at heart.

Doctors and nurses are under even more pressure to conform than parents. Questioning procedure and protocol can be very expensive for them. Peer pressure is taken to a whole new level. The ranks are so tight that even if a doctor is just flat out bad, his peers will clean up his messes before they will expose him. Even if ACOG's recommendations lack all common sense, they follow them. The reward is that they in turn are supported if they make a mistake. However, there is a difference in making an honest mistake, and true malpractice. If there was less tolerance for bad care within the ranks, parents might not be forced to take legal action as their only perceived recourse.

Fear for doctors and nurses includes the fear of litigation, in addition to a fear of birth and of being ostracized. There are financial rewards in sticking together. There are also financial rewards for routine use of technology.

For a long time I wanted to minimize financial incentive for maintaining the status quo when it means mothers and babies are put at risk. Conversations with doctors themselves who insist that money and power are at the root of the abysmal conditions we now face have convinced me that it is a reward that motivates at least a few.

Doctors (and at least one certified nurse-midwife I've talked to) have explained to me how the money and fear of litigation create a sort of circular logic that allows patients (and lawyers) to practice medicine.

They insist that they only do the things they do because the women demand it. If they didn't do what the women wanted, then the women would go elsewhere (taking their purses with them). By not doing something that someone else would do, they stand to lose a great deal (of money and acceptance both) if they follow the science instead of 'standard of care.' Standard of care means, basically, what everyone else is doing.

We see this with antibiotic use also, which has led us to a place where antibiotic resistant organisms run rampant. (FDA, 2011; CDC, 2012) But mainly, we see it in very limited situations.

If I went to a doctor and demanded Vicodin for common stress headaches, I'm guessing I'd be hard pressed to find a doctor who would buy into that.

128

What if I went in and demanded an appendectomy because I have an irrational fear of the pain and possible death of a ruptured appendix? Would I be able to find a doctor who would take it out 'just in case?'

My guess is that doctors would explain the actual incidence of ruptured appendixes, would only do appendectomies if clinical signs and symptoms were present, and maybe even educate the general public about their misconceptions.

Most in what we call the 'helping professions' went into it to help people. They believe they are helping. To think otherwise would be painful, so denial is useful in avoiding emotional pain. That makes total sense. Change is painful sometimes. Avoiding pain is a reward.

Another reward is one that I didn't think of until it was pointed out to me by someone in a helping profession; being able to rush in and save the day is appealing to many. Maybe not consciously, but heroism addiction is easy to plug into. What a feeling of power to think that an event could not happen safely without out them. Certainly, we all like to feel needed. It's easy to see how seductive this reward might be.

As for ACOG, what is their motivation for making recommendations that fly in the face of common sense and decency, not to mention science? It doesn't seem to be for the sake of mothers and babies, that's for sure.

Lawyers
In the age of the frivolous lawsuits, lawyers could do much to change the system if they refused to sue doctors for being human so that doctors would not have to practice defensive medicine.

Media

The media reflects society's core beliefs. What sells is the bottom line and what sells is drama, disaster, blood, death and rescue. The media portrays birth the way it does because we are watching it and they are making money.

In conclusion, while our maternity care system doesn't 'work' in that it produces the best outcomes or deliver affordable care, it does reward each participant in some way, shape or form, recognizable or not.

Are you on the path of least resistance? What would happen if we all did one thing different?

What if television and movies started portraying birth as joyful, easy and even funny without relying on the pain card?

What if good doctors, practicing evidence-based care, refused to support the sub-standard practice of their peers?

What if lawyers refused to try cases in which the doctor did nothing intentionally wrong?

What if parents demanded respect and became informed consumers?

What if we come back to common sense?

What if…

Aside from our motivating factors, we must examine some of our 'tendencies' as well.

We are said to be the 'me' generation…the 'now' generation. We've heard ourselves referred to as a 'feel good' society. We want it, we want it when we want it, and we don't feel we need to work to get it.

We don't tend to look past our own noses, let alone seven generations ahead.

If a person is currently in pain and looking for relief in the moment, that is a much more urgent consideration than oxygen deprivation in the neonate due to narcotics...that may or may not contribute to special education classes for a child 7 years from now. Feeling good now is a powerful motivator. (And may well be how the baby was conceived in the first place!) Consequences affecting ourselves, or our children, down the road seem remote possibilities, abstract and not very compelling, if faced with inevitable suffering right now. Is suffering inevitable in birth? It is only if you want to believe it into being.

So, what are the real reasons stopping you from creating the best birth possible for you? Is there a social pay-off in being able to share the same 'war story' as your friends? Is it to avoid emotional pain of rejection, or unreasonable fear of the expectation of unbearable physical pain?

If you fail to identify and understand your motivators others can manipulate you with them. It happens everyday. Women have been coerced into non-medically indicated interventions with their unconscious motivators with such tactics as being asked, "Am I the only one who cares about this baby?" or "Do you really want to kill this baby and put yourself at risk?"

Parents can be on the giving end of manipulative tactics as well. The word 'malpractice' comes to mind.

Nurses (and some female doctors...the highest rates of cesareans being nurses, doctors, and doctor's wives) who either didn't labor at all or labored with drugs have been known to tell women who don't want drugs, "Oh, come on! Don't be a martyr!" even when the mother is quite comfortable and coping well.

Free yourself from the tools of manipulation by knowing your own system of motivation. If you are knowledgeable, if you know you are making a decision from a place of confidence, these power plays will have no effect on you.

One last thing that must be mentioned is that parents would not knowingly consent to worthless and expensive testing or birth technology, much less potentially harmful intervention. Yet, the premise of this work thus far is that consent is given millions of times everyday, and that current obstetrical management is harmful and unnecessary.

Motivating factors aside, would fear override good judgment if parents had all the facts? Do they have 'balanced' information or is their fear and lack of unbiased pregnancy and childbirth information played upon? Know what is normal for you and this won't happen. I had a client who had a caregiver that tried to manipulate her into some testing by saying accusingly, "Your hemoglobin has dropped to 12!" as if was a catastrophe. If you know that 12 is within normal limits late in pregnancy or what your hemoglobin has been at for the last few weeks, this tactic won't work on you. Women have been coerced into a cesarean because "your baby's heart rate had dropped to 120...he's in distress and we need to get him out of there" when 120 beats per minute is well within normal limits.

Mainstream childbirth information is held and dispersed, for the most part, by a self-perpetuating system. There is other information out there, but you must seek it out. It doesn't take mountains of scientific literature to break this cycle, though it is plentiful for those who want to avail themselves of it. A few questions can do the job. Start with an attitude of "Show me the evidence!"

In pregnancy or birth, when an intervention or test is suggested, ask:

- What does this test for, specifically?
- Where can I find further information on this condition?

- What personal risk factors indicate I may have/develop this condition/problem?
- What signs or symptoms indicate I may have this problem? Please supply me with normal parameters so that I may see where I am in regard to 'normal.'
- How accurate is this test? What is the rate of false positives? How reproducible is it?
- What are the possible risks of this test? (Beware of a 'none' response!)
- Could this test lead to others? What are they?
- (repeat all above questions for each subsequent test before consent)
- If this problem/condition is detected, can it be fixed? How?
- What is the incidence of spontaneous improvement of this condition?
- What is the success rate of intervention for this condition?
- Is this condition/problem considered a variable by some practitioners, or is it always considered a complication?
- How might someone who sees it as a variable proceed?
- What if we do nothing? (Simpkin, n.d.)

An example might be routine ultrasound to rule out ectopic pregnancy.

Ectopic pregnancy is on the rise, and it is a leading cause of pregnancy related death. (Saftlas, Lawson, Atrash, nd) This is very scary, right?

Well, the death rate for ectopic pregnancy is roughly the same as death from an auto accident for women aged 15 to 35; something to be aware of, but probably not something you think about each time you hop in the car to go get a quart of milk.

There are certain identifiable risk factors that can lead to ectopic pregnancy. Routinely testing a high-risk population is probably prudent use of technology.

Ultrasound is undoubtedly effective in detecting this condition. Is it safe? There is some evidence that suggests we should use it sparingly because there are possible risks. (Midwifery Today, nd.) Is there an alternative? How about telling women what early signs and symptoms are and making sure they know the importance in contacting their caregiver, reserving testing for high-risk women?

> "THERE IS NOTHING EITHER GOOD OR BAD, BUT THINKING MAKES IT SO."
> WILLIAM SHAKESPEARE

Another example might be premature labor. It is a complication dreaded by both caregiver and by parent alike. Parents, faced with the threat of pregnancy loss, are understandably desperate to save the life of their child.

Caring practitioners obviously don't want to see the parent endure the painful process of loss either, but in a litigious society such as our own, we must also recognize the imperative to give the appearance that every attempt has been made to avoid such loss, even if the futility of such an attempt is well known by the medical professional. Modern medicine has tried very hard to reduce the number of premature deliveries, but sadly, very few of the current standard practices are able to stop a true premature birth. According to the March of Dimes (MOD, 2010), the incidence of premature delivery, before 37 weeks gestation, has increased by 36% since the early '80s.

Does this increase suggest that mothers are becoming less healthy, despite numerous campaigns to improve the heath of mothers and babies? While that may seem to be the case at first glance, it may not actually be so. There are other causes to prematurity that are often ignored, including preventable prematurity due to increasing numbers of vaginal infections, for instance. Also to be considered are cases of premature labor being diagnosed and treated where it does not exist as previously mentioned, as well as a high number of inductions often resulting in unnecessary cesareans because the ultrasound was wrong on dates or baby's size...a common occurrence.

The March of Dimes is concerned about these iotrogenic (doctor caused) cases of preventable prematurity. (ibid.)

Consider, the mother who is expecting twins, who is told throughout her pregnancy that twins always come early. She takes excellent care of herself and goes past her doctors predicted six-week early delivery date. She goes past 34 weeks. Then she makes it to 36 weeks.

Her doctor tells her that she needs to be induced because 'the babies aren't growing.' Two babies nearly 7 pounds each are forced from the womb (not bad for early twins that 'weren't growing'...had she remained pregnant she might have had 8 lb. babies, laying waste to the claim that 'twins are always small'), and their birth will be listed as premature, strengthening the argument that 'everyone knows twins come early.'

Certain obstetrical complications tend to fall into and out of favor. Premature labor does really exist in a small number of pregnancies. However, alarmingly, many women are being diagnosed and treated with drugs and protocol that aren't even effective for the true condition of prematurity, much less where it does not exist.

Remember Chloe's story? Not all similar situations end up with healthy babies and empowered mothers.

Most often the faulty diagnosis of premature labor examined here is made via unnecessary routine and potentially dangerous (Lenihan,1984; McDuffie,1992) vaginal exams and superfluous electronic fetal monitoring (EFM) devices in the office. Mom is not told that neither provides useful information in that setting. Never mind that they definition of pre-term labor includes contractions that get longer, stronger and closer together while opening the cervix. Is it reasonable to assume that this kind of progression could be determined by one routine internal digital exam and EFM per month, even per week? Not really...much closer observation would be required.

Nevertheless, Mom is so alarmed at the possibility of losing her baby that she often isn't thinking critically. She's willing to do anything to save her baby.

She also probably doesn't know that even if she is dilated a couple of centimeters, it can be completely normal.

So, the mom's cervix is sewn up (cerclage) or she given terbutaline and put on bed rest. She's so grateful that her doctor 'caught' this, of course, yet there is more she doesn't know. She doesn't know that in study after study, terbutaline doesn't do a thing to stop true premature labor. (FDA, 2011) She also doesn't know that this drug isn't approved by the FDA for pregnancy, labor, delivery or lactation, or that the FDA warns that it should not be used to stop or slow contractions because "Serious adverse reactions may occur after administration of terbutaline sulfate to women in labor." (AIMS, nd.) The pregnancy continues (because it would have anyway) but there is no way to prove that it wouldn't have, so the assumption is that the only reason it did was because of the efforts of the doctor.

Because the drug definitely crosses the placenta, baby experiences the same thing that mom is, including heart rate accelerations. If the mom is unable to eat from the nausea, the combination of not being able to keep anything down, the effect on her already taxed liver, and the high blood pressure, she will quite likely develop complications that were completely preventable. Up to this point, very similar to Chloe.

Now mother and baby need to be 'saved.' Mom will be induced. If she really had been experiencing premature labor this would be easy, since she was on her way already, right? Except that in this case, she wasn't in premature labor. The induction doesn't work on this hard, high, closed cervix.

Since many inductions start with a prostaglandin ripening agent, rupture of the membranes and pitocin or misoprosol (Cytotc), an ulcer drug and chemical abortion agent, again, not only not approved by the FDA for this use, but known to cause a number of complications, (FDA, 2009) the mom is on a clock. If she doesn't deliver in 24 hours or less, she will be told she must have a cesarean. Of course, because her water has been broken and fingers have been inside her constantly since she arrived, there is a high probability that she will get a hospital acquired infection and the cesarean may be warranted. Although again...preventable and caused, not encountered. This woman will get an unnecessary cesarean and be eternally grateful that her doctor 'saved' her, completely unaware that all of it was avoidable.

Remember that premature labor is an actual medical condition. So how does a mother know if she really has it and does need medical assistance or if something else is going on? How is real premature labor diagnosed? What causes it?

How can a mother reduce her chances of going into labor too soon, and if it does happen to her, what are the effective treatments? What treatments, (besides terbutaline) have been shown to be ineffective, and what are their risks?

According to the March of Dimes, twenty-five percent of preterm, low birth weight cases occur without any known risk factors. Prediction of this sector is nearly impossible. When it occurs, blame must not be placed at the feet of the practitioner who is treading a very fine line between prudent use of technology that could save a life, and inappropriate use of technology in the name of 'defensive medicine' that could cost lives.

Prevention is the best medicine when it comes to lowering the rate of prematurity. Most premature labor could be avoided if mothers improved their health by quitting smoking, not using alcohol, eating better and preventing urinary tract infections. Sometimes the importance of optimizing health through nutrition is not made very clear, as caregivers face being labeled 'judgmental' for trying to encourage mothers to stop smoking or for pointing out that negative behavior choices could have life-long ramifications. Unfortunately, those that cave into political correctness around the issues may then be sued when a baby is premature because honesty and sparing the parents the emotional and financial hardships (conservatively projected at $500,000 for the life of the child) of raising a baby born prematurely might have made a mother feel guilty, which could have lost them a client.

Mothers need to be properly nourished for placental health. Most mothers have complete control over what they put in their bodies. Admittedly not every mother does, and those that do don't always what will remain in their bodies if they experience nausea and vomiting. In these instances moms need to remember to control what can be controlled, work with what can't, or accept what is if that is the only option. A baby who is not getting the essential requirements for optimal growth and well-being is more likely to be born prematurely so as a society, it is in our best interest to help these women. Nutrition is also vitally important for the health of mom. Dr. Tom Brewer has done extensive work on the effect of nutrition and pre-eclampsia/toxemia.

Similarly, smoking damages the placenta in a number of ways. Carbon monoxide replaces a great deal of oxygen that should be going to the placenta and baby. Because cyanide, arsenic, nicotine and countless other toxins also pollute the fetal environment, the placenta might grow over more of the surface of the uterus seeking oxygen, or, it might fail to grow large enough to meet the needs of the baby because it isn't getting enough oxygen. Small dead areas called "infarcs" are more common in smokers, areas that cannot deliver nutrients and oxygen to the baby...which is why smokers' babies are smaller than babies born to non-smoking mothers and prematurity is more common in smokers.

Infections are another cause of pre-mature labor. Routine vaginal exams in pregnancy serve no purpose. It has been theorized that excessive use of this pointless ritual contributes to premature labor and premature rupture of the membranes by introducing germs to the cervix on the examiners glove. Even sterile technique isn't truly sterile. In any case, a pelvic exam without medical indication tells the caregiver nothing. A woman can be dilated to 2 centimeters at 34 weeks and still be pregnant past her 'due date.' Likewise, a woman can be 'high, firm and closed' and have a three-hour labor at 41 weeks.

Dehydration often causes premature contractions. Mothers must take in at least ten 8-ounce glasses of water a day, not including other liquids in the equation. In hot weather she needs more. Insufficient water intake is also a factor in bladder infections in pregnancy, which can cause pre-term labor.

Multiples are often expected to be premature in the medical model, but is that expectation a given? No. Midwives attending well-nourished mothers of multiples often not only have moms who reach their 'due date', but go 'over due' to deliver healthy babies of normal weight. With twins, it may very well be the expectation of the caregiver (thus, the management of the pregnancy) that is the biggest factor in early delivery of twins, excluding the rare medical abnormality.

Avoidance of all non-medically indicated prenatal testing reduces the chance of being misdiagnosed or over-diagnosed, a subject which Henci Goer has extensively explored and documented in *Obstetric Myths verses Research Realities*.

Establishing communication with your caregiver about the medical applicability, risks and benefits to any-and-all interventions, not just in pregnancy but through the birth, is vitally important. Any doctor who is practicing evidence based care will welcome this exchange and be pleased that you would like to take more responsibility in your care. A doctor who becomes angry that you would like more information, defensive that you would require evidence of efficacy or condescending toward your efforts to be knowledgeable is waving a big red flag.

What's a parent to do if, by some fluke of nature or circumstance, premature labor has become their reality? (Enkin et al, 1995)

Interventions that have been shown to be of questionable or no value:

Home uterine activity monitoring
Bed rest
Repeated vaginal exams
Ultrasound assessment of cervical length

Interventions that have been shown to be of questionable or no value and which may pose significant risk:

Terbutaline
Magnesium Sulphate (although this has been shown to arrest uterine contractions in women who are not actually in preterm labor...exactly the situation in this example just provided...but with serious side effects)
Cervical cerclage

Interventions that may help but not without significant risk:

Prostaglandin inhibitors
Ritodrine

Interventions that seem to help without significant risk and warrant further investigation:

Calcium supplementation
Progestogens
Antimicrobial agents (antibiotics)

Interventions with insufficient data to warrant regular use:

Diazoxide
Oxytocin antagonists

Significantly effective with no risk:

Hypnosis (Brown & Murphy, 1999)

What is the very best way to avoid being treated for a condition that doesn't exist? For starters, see a midwife or holistic general practitioner in pregnancy instead of surgical specialist like an obstetrician. If an underlying medical condition dictates that you must see an expert in pathology (illness), such as an OB/GYN, initiate dialog early about appropriate birth technology specific to your situation. Learn about what you can do to be healthier and how you can best assist your caregiver in your treatment.

Don't be afraid to get second opinions or change caregivers if yours is not treating you respectfully and helping you to learn about your condition. People treat us as we allow. If you don't speak up, you play a part in the creation of your own experience.

Let's look at just one labor intervention as another illustration:

The policy of fasting in labor and an IV are two interventions that go hand in hand. The rationale given is that anything could go wrong at any minute, requiring surgery. If that were to happen they need to be able to 'have a vein open.' Also, if surgery becomes necessary, the stomach should be empty because one complication of general anesthesia is that it can cause vomiting.

This all sounds reasonable to the parents, after all, it is for their safety. But is it?

An IV is a good idea if the mother is vomiting constantly, unable to keep food and fluids down. Obviously, if a woman is planning surgery, an IV is required.

An EMT can find a vein to place an IV in a car crash victim who has been bleeding out into a ditch until their arrival.

Why can't highly trained nurses attending a pregnant woman find a vein in an emergency in which medical personnel have been no more than a few steps away?

Pregnancy complications rarely happen, but when they do, there are often indications that something is going wrong long before.

Any time the skin is pierced, as in with an IV, there is risk of infection. In the hospital, that means super germs that can be fatal. IV fluids can dilute the mother's own birth-regulating hormones and comfort hormones, which means artificial ones are more likely to be required. (Many women, upon requesting their birth records, have discovered easy access to a vein allowed these artificial substances to be administered without their consent.)

If a mother is allowed to eat and drink as she desires in labor, dehydration is rarely a problem, providing she is not vomiting everything she takes in. Most mothers are not allowed food due to the unlikely event she should require surgery. Note the circular logic of the simple act of placing an IV into a laboring woman increasing her chances of needing surgery.

It is true if general anesthesia is incorrectly administered it can cause vomiting that could theoretically be inhaled into the lungs. However, general anesthesia is rarely used since the advent of the epidural, even in emergency situations. IF general anesthesia is used, IF it is administered incorrectly and IF a mother aspirates the contents of the stomach…the acidic contents of an empty stomach are actually more damaging to the lungs than easily digestible food. Thus, it would make sense to just allow women to eat and drink. But upon discovery that the acidic contents are more damaging, what is the obstetrical solution? Give antacids, of course!

Asking questions and testing the validity of the answers with good old-fashioned critical thinking skills can reveal the underlying unsound nature of most routine intervention.

142

CHAPTER 6
Mother Nature

Fairy tale births do exist! (I'll keep repeating that until you believe me!)

Creating a wonderful birth requires a combination of good decision-making, decent circumstances and a little bit of luck, in that order.

If you want a safe and satisfying birth, the odds are overwhelmingly in your favor to have it…if you seriously set out to have it. Nature has designed it that way. The way to keep it that way is to keep it close to the original design, which has worked as long as humans have been populating the earth.

We know this design works because the healthy mothers who follow the plan are the ones of which other mothers are so envious. In fact, envy, one of those lenses that colors what we see, prompts the unhappy mothers into believing that the happy mothers are lying or, at the very least, just lucky.

Not so.

Keep in mind that while we have the blueprint for happy healthy mothers and babies, there will be a few, a very few, who do everything outlined and still be unhappy…just as there are a few who will do everything antithetical to a fairy tale birth and still be quite happy with no unfortunate results.

Remember this book is not about 'right' or 'not right.' If you were induced and had an epidural with no negative consequences to your baby or yourself, that's fantastic! Not all women who have medicated births will have jaundiced babies, difficulty breastfeeding or challenging postpartum recovery resulting from the cascade of interventions that usually follow. There are mothers who intended to have home births that later were not happy with their choices and so condemn all home birth.

The elements of a great birth are what we scientifically know will result in the best possible birth most of the time. The conclusions are based on years of statistical analysis and matched populations. You are not a statistic. The best I can do is to tell you what joyful mothers do and have done. If you make the same choices you will probably get the same results. If you make the same choices that unhappy mothers get, you will probably get the same results. That is just common sense.

By now, you should be able to see that options you didn't think pertained to you are really quite possible for you.

Remember the elements of the safest, gentlest births, resulting in healthy babies and happy moms (Stewart, 1981):

Good nutrition
Skilled Midwifery
Home birth with skilled midwives
Natural Childbirth
Breastfeeding

Good nutrition:

I have heard women complain about the nutritional ideals put forth by other books. The food necessary to grow healthy babies is not what many of us are used to eating.

That doesn't change the fact that we grow our babies with every single substance we put into our bodies. These babies will have those bodies for the rest of their lives. You will care for those bodies for the next 18 years. Trust me, mothering is hard enough without starting a child's life encumbered by asthma or prematurity.

What does good nutrition encompass? Simplified, it means eating nutritious food and avoiding junk. If you used to eat white bread, eat whole wheat while you are pregnant. If you've never eaten organic, make some of your produce organic. If you used to drink soda, drink water.

If you normally eat a lot of empty calories, ask yourself if what you are about to put in your mouth contributes to your baby's heath or is a detriment to it.

If you would be inclined to drink juice, eat the fruit. If you can't stand vegetables, drink vegetable juice. If you prefer 'cheese products,' choose real cheese instead. If you don't like milk, eat yogurt.

There are several things to remember about diet that are more important than others.

Proteins are the building blocks of your baby. Not only is it important to ingest more protein (80-100 grams a day) to build your baby, but it's important in avoiding pre-eclampsia as well, according to practitioners who follow Dr. Tom Brewer's guidelines for healthy pregnancy.

Adequate water, calcium and salt intake are also important. The pregnant body produces about 50% more blood to meet the demands of the placenta to nourish the growing baby. To do this, the body needs more fluid. Incidentally, more fluid means that there will be dilution of the components of the blood, which is why hemoglobin levels appear to fall. A contracted blood volume, for example from dehydration, would mean that substances are elevated in the blood stream, which is one reason why premature labor can result from dehydration.

In any case, I visited one hospital where all of the babies in the nursery that day were delivered via cesarean surgeries due to pre-eclampsia.

I was shocked, because in the previous months as a midwife's apprentice, pre-eclampsia was never ever seen once.

Pre-eclampsia is a very serious disorder in pregnancy. The medical establishment still maintains that they don't know what causes it and that it cannot be prevented. I've read theories that it has to do with everything from multiple partners to heredity, and the latest, that the body makes too much of a certain protein.

Dr. Tom Brewer's extensive research on the topic suggests that protein, calcium and adequate salt intake are critical in avoiding illness.

Midwives using his information almost never see pre-eclampsia unless there is some pre-existing underlying liver compromise. Dr. Brewer's work is available online. (Brewer, n.d.)

Babies need to grow on actual food, not prenatal vitamins. While vitamins can pick up some of the slack of an otherwise lacking food program, it's really best to eat the foods, which have the necessary extra calories needed to sustain a healthy pregnancy.

Prenatal vitamins cause some women more grief than they're worth if they contain ferrous sulfinate, which most prescribed prenatal vitamins do. Women report nausea and constipation. Nausea can lead to problems like low blood sugar, which perpetuates the cycle of nausea and vomiting. Constipation can lead to hemorrhoids, at the very least. This is because the body does not absorb ferrous sulfinate very well. Because only about 30% of what is ingested is absorbed they are manufactured with more than the minimum daily requirement for pregnant women.

There are products available with the more easily absorbed ferrous gluconate. Still, food sources are best. Iron is important in pregnancy because you are helping your baby build a storehouse of available iron until he or she produces his or her own, long after birth.

146

Also, iron is important in the production of hemoglobin, which helps your red blood cells carry oxygen to your baby.

Sugar is a huge problem in our culture. Sugar consumption (not only in the form obvious sugar, but in the form of foods so processed that they break down quickly into sugar) is responsible for high type-2 diabetes rates and obesity. In pregnancy, sugar and insulin work differently, which can create significant problems.

While babies are built on protein, they grow on glucose...sugar. In order to produce healthy, plump babies, insulin production changes so that sugar is more available to the growing baby. Of course, this design maximized growth when early humans ate whole foods. Now, it works against us.

Currently, scientists are researching the theory that foods with a high glycemic index are the cause of many health problems, such as obesity and heart disease, within the general population. It would stand to reason that the solution to insulin/sugar problems in pregnancy would be to avoid foods with a high glycemic index in the first place.

Another danger is if all that sugar makes babies 'macrosomatic'...big. This is where the medical establishment's fear of 'big babies' comes from. Some big babies may result in shoulder dystocia, meaning the baby gets stuck, though one has to wonder just what the natural incidence is and what is due to mismanagement since midwives regularly help mothers birth babies in the 8 to 10 pound range or bigger with no problem.

If mom has been ingesting large quantities of sugar, baby may also have hypoglycemic episodes after the birth, when the sugar supply is cut off. Sugar water was given to babies after birth to avoid this very thing. (Though now it continues to be routine for babies who are not showing signs of hypoglycemia.) If a mother has not been a sugar hound or isn't a true diabetic, and the baby is allowed to nurse to his or her hearts content after the birth, sugar water isn't necessary. Not only that, but bottles of sugar water can set up breastfeeding challenges resulting in horrible pain for the mother and early weaning.

When I speak of big babies here, I mean over 10 lb...not 8 or 9 lb. as medically minded care providers assert is 'too big'. Unnecessary cesarean sections for CPD (head/pelvis disproportion) are common for babies predicted (via ultrasound) to be too big to birth but turn out average or smaller.

Over the years, many women in my own classes and those of my colleagues have consented to a cesarean because they were told their babies were huge (8 or 9 lb.) only to have a 6 lb. peanut-baby surgically delivered. Ultrasound is not a good predictor of baby's weight, it's only accurate to within 2 lb. either way...for a total of a 4 lb. range. Neither does it 'change' your due date. How many times does your conception date change?

Eight or nine pound babies are healthy and most mothers, barring a pelvic abnormality, can birth this size baby just fine. Bigger babies can actually be easier to birth than smaller because positional complications are not seen as often.

What people don't often think about is that nature has an interest in seeing that as many offspring as possible survive birth. We don't make babies too big to birth without some sort of outside variable. If a 4'10" mother makes a baby with a 6'6" father, her baby might be too big to fit through her pelvis.

If a mother grows her baby on a truckload of sugar, her baby might be too big to fit through her pelvis. If a mother was malnourished as a child and her bones did not develop properly, or her pelvis was damaged in some sort of accident, her baby might not fit. Most of the time, however, our wise bodies grow babies just the right size to be born through the body in which they were made and grown.

Not seemingly related to nutrition, but absolutely related to healthy babies and birth, is smoking. Now is the time to take charge of this monkey on your back if you are a smoking mother. Smoking robs the body of B vitamins, vitamin C and others essential to healthy pregnancy. (Cogswell, Weisberg & Spong, 2003)

Skillful midwifery:

Skillful midwifery can mean certified professional midwives, certified nurse midwives or traditional birth attendants. It may also mean a doctor working within the midwifery model of care.

The midwifery model sees birth as a healthy, normal social event instead of a medical disaster waiting to happen. The care reflects that mind set.

Pregnancies are monitored with minimal invasiveness. Baseline readings are taken to establish 'normal' for a given woman. At a minimum, blood pressure, urine, fundal height, fetal heart tones and sometimes hemoglobin are assessed. The emotional and social needs of the mother are evaluated, with referral to support networks where indicated. Each visit will usually last at least an hour.

The mother is also counseled in the importance of good nutrition, with assistance in formulating a program that works with the mother's own preferences. If something is askew, the midwife refers to a physician to investigate further...where doctors are willing to work with the midwives. Midwives prefer to offer collaborative models where continuity of care can be established. Unfortunately, in some areas their efforts are not reciprocated by other professionals.

To see how a fear-based paradigm differs from a evidence-based, safety-focused, mother-centered paradigm, consider the following:

Say a midwife has a client who comes early in pregnancy. The midwife refuses to take her unless she stops smoking and gets a back-up physician.

At subsequent visits, the client first a.) says she forgot to set up an appointment with her doctor for blood work b.) says she missed an appointment with her doctor because she forgot and c.) says the doctor won't take her because she's planning a home birth with a midwife.

Throughout, the mother's baselines (blood pressure, fetal growth & movement, urine dipstick readings, fetal heart tones, etc.) are all within normal limits.

Since the mother's last birth was within the last couple of years, with the same partner, the midwife agrees that if she gets her records and blood work from last time, at least they'll have a starting reference point. Intuitively, the midwife is uncomfortable, even though all clinical observations are reassuring.

By the 20-week appointment, after several more maternal lies, omissions and discovery that the mother has not quit smoking, the midwife can no longer ignore her intuition. She dismisses the client with a registered letter, explaining that without trust and responsible action on the part of the mother, birth at home is not a safe option. The choices made by the mother are putting her at risk for certain complications that make the hospital the only safe option. The midwife gives the names of three caregivers chosen from the phone book…her only recourse because all of the doctors have refused to meet with her to discuss providing continuity of care for her clients.

Months later, the midwife runs into the woman who tells her that the birth ended up requiring emergency assistance due to placental abruption and hemorrhage…the exact complications the midwife suspected might happen and knew could not be handled safely at home.

In a system concerned primarily with the safety of mother and baby, this midwife would be congratulated recognizing her limits, referring to an appropriate professional and probably saving a mother's life and/or that of her baby.

In a provider-centered system, the doctors are angry that they have to deal with a sick person. Petty and retaliatory measures are sure to follow. These could include everything from behavior bordering on restraint-of-trade, to making it impossible for the midwife and her family to receive medical care in their own community. There are even many cases of criminal charges leading to jail for midwives with better outcomes than the doctors that instigated the charges!

Midwives are trained to care for 'normal,' recognizing abnormal. They are trained in emergency procedures in the event of time-sensitive complications.

Where the doctors and midwives work together, in the rare event of a medical emergency at a freestanding birth center or home, the 'decision to incision' time for a cesarean is about the same as it would be for a woman actually in the hospital, where she may have to wait for her surgeon to get to her.

Home birth

Home birth as safe as hospital birth, under normal circumstances, not only due to the temptation in the hospital to inappropriately use the technology at hand, but for biological reasons.

The mother is immune to all of the germs in her own home. The most foreign thing there would be the care provider that came to assist her. Because the mother has immunity to everything in her environment, so does her baby. Hospital acquired infections cause a large number of the thousands of deaths due to medical mistakes. Why would we want to expose healthy mothers and fragile newborns to these 'super bugs' intentionally?

Next, the mammalian 'birthing brain' functions best in one's own 'nest.' Mothers are less likely to produce adrenaline, the fight or flight hormone, if the sights, smells and sounds around her are familiar. Adrenaline is counterproductive to oxytocin, the mother's own naturally produced birthing hormone.

Because mom is more relaxed, births tend to be shorter and more comfortable at home. Mom can eat and drink to keep her strength up, can move around at will and can utilize water to her advantage by getting in the tub if she feels like it.

At least part of the reason that Mongan Method HypnoBirthing® helps women in the hospital achieve shorter, safer, more comfortable birth is because the self-hypnosis intentionally sets up a sort of 'cocoon' for mom. An environment perceived to be safe is one of the four requirements of eliciting the 'relaxation response.'

The 'relaxation response' is the term Dr. Herbert Benson gave the opposite of the 'fight or flight' response in his Harvard studies on the effects of stress on the body. His findings are applicable to simplifying the birthing process. (Benson, 1976; 1985)

Studies have shown that births where the relaxation response is engaged...home births and births using self-hypnosis or similar techniques most notably, are as safe as, or safer than hospital birth, with fewer birth related injuries to both mother and child. (Schauble, Werner, Rai & Martin, 1998; Harmon, Hynan & Tyre, 1990).

Natural Birth

Avoiding unnecessary interventions is perhaps the most important element to a safe birth. The technology was created to help sick or injured pregnant women. It is helpful to those women. Applied indiscriminately and routinely to all birthing women, it creates many the problems we see in birth today. But we need it for the sick and injured!

Interventions may seem trivial in and of themselves, but they lead down a dangerous path that results in disruption to the essential hormonal balance and natural physiological systems needed for comfortable, safe birth.

In the absence of the medical indication for which they were developed, birth interventions are at best worthless, at worst, harmful.

None of what modern women view as "normal" birth...IV, medications, laying flat on the back, monitors, catheters, episiotomies/stitches, babies whisked off to warming tables, a room full of doctors and nurses...has anything to do with what should be normal birth the way nature intended.

Truly normal birth...natural birth...is gentle, loving and peaceful. It is an intimate event between the parents and a new being their love created. The organs and hormones that made the baby are the very same ones involved in getting the baby out. In fact, natural birth often sounds and looks very much like love-making. The same things that would disrupt a sexual encounter disrupt the birthing process.

Nature provides us with many mechanisms to be comfortable in birth. I've even seen orgasmic birth. I believe it is not birth itself that creates pain, but the fear/tension/pain cycle. Sometimes, our bodies use pain to communicate a need. On occasion, some abnormality causes pain. Pain itself does not have to be inherent in birth.

I bring this up before the chapter on pain because we now have a 90% national epidural rate in some places. Virtually all women birthing in the hospital have some drug, even if it isn't an epidural.

All drugs tamper with the delicate balance nature provided, by a number of different mechanisms. All drugs affect the baby, some by prolonging labor, some by restricting oxygen, some by hindering the reflexes meant to assist baby's transition from the womb to the room.

Maybe short term, maybe long term, maybe obviously or subtly, but they all affect the baby.

Pain relievers and narcotics disrupt the feedback loop for the mothers birthing hormones. These reach the baby and are hard for the baby's immature liver to process. They make babies sleepy, sometimes for weeks, and complicate the nursing process.

Pitocin fools the mother's body into thinking it doesn't have to make its own oxytocin, which can lead to hemorrhage. As a synthetic oxytocin, it blocks endorphins which increases pain. (Buckley, 2002) Contractions stimulated by pitocin are abnormally long and strong, which increases stress on the baby. Severe postpartum depression has been linked to both pitocin use and a decrease in the mothers own production of oxytocin.

Natural labor and birthing result in dramatic brain chemistry changes in both mother and baby. Bonding is not just a function of proximity, though that is important. Bonding includes a complex interchange of chemical messengers that actually change the brain structure of mother and baby to create a symbiotic partnership for survival. (ibid.)

There are medical reasons to use both pitocin and epidurals on occasion, but women are choosing both thinking there is no risk to either...often because that is what they are told. Months later they wonder why they feel strangely disconnected from their children. The erroneous assumption has been made that bonding is a myth. It is absolutely a reality! It's just been sabotaged in so many mothers in America.

If birth didn't work, if nature made a mistake, if birth were so dangerous, could we have survived in such huge numbers?

Hospitals and doctors, the currently assumed factors in safe birth, didn't even enter the picture until about 90-100 years ago! In fact, when birth was first moved to hospitals (for the sake of caregiver's

154

convenience, not for safety as is often presumed) maternal mortality (death) rates increased. (Gibson, 2006) Dr. Semmelweis recognized that this high rate of 'childbed fever' was due to the practice of doctors moving from cadavers to birthing mothers without washing their hands, but it would be another 50 years before his 'radical' ideas would be met with anything but derision by his peers.

Far more significant in the reduction of maternal and infant death are the contributing factors of improved sanitation, antibiotics, birth control, better nutrition and disease management.

Natural birth is important, not just one choice between two equals. There are reasons to educate yourself about the benefits to you and your baby.

Breastfeeding

Babies aren't actually 'done' when mom's belly button timer pops. Human babies are born before they are actually ready to be out here on their own. They are born more helpless than other mammals because they have to be. Human babies may be born earlier than other primates so that their relatively large heads, containing bigger brains, fit well through their mother's upright pelvis.

All mammals, animals with mammary glands, give birth to live babies that need to be close to their mothers until they no longer need the milk made just for them, specifically…at least two years, but much longer where nutritious food is scarce. Human babies' brains grow at an astonishing rate in the first two years of life. Mother's milk gives their brains the building blocks to grow bigger brains with more neurological connections. Yes, that means higher IQ, but there is another brain size connection as well.

Researchers have studied children with ADHD who have smaller brains. (Greene, 2002) They thought that it might have been caused by the medications prescribed to control the disorder.

There is now data that suggests that is not the case.

ADHD seems to be a mild form of autism, (Kennedy, 2002) which has increased by an alarming amount in recent years. (ARI, 2012) While ultrasound exposure (Robison, 2012) medications or interventions in birth (Autism Today, nd.), early cord clamping (Morley, nd.) and vaccines (NVIC, 2012) have all been implicated in this rise, it is very likely that lack of mother's milk is also a contributing factor. (Schultz, Klonoff-Cohen, Wingard, Akshoomoff, Macera, Ji, & Bacher, 2006)

I have been asked in classes "If a mother isn't going to breastfeed, what is the closest thing to human mother's milk?" There is nothing like breast milk. That is not a judgment of mothers who don't feed their babies the milk made especially for them. It is a fact.

There are proteins in mother's milk that build your baby's brain. These proteins cannot be duplicated in a lab. There are living components to mother's milk that help babies ward off illness until their own immune system develops that cannot be duplicated. The composition of a mother's milk will change from feeding to feeding, based on her own infants needs.

The physical ailments that have increased dramatically with the advent of bottle-feeding are commonly discussed. One writer (writing anonymously, for she said she feared the 'nipple-Nazis'...though she did not specify what she feared) in a popular pregnancy magazine questioned just how much better breastfeeding was. The numbers on the differences childhood illnesses wasn't enough proof for her, it seems. In any case, she decided to focus on the bonding issue and declared that if bottle-feeding really was inferior to mother-feeding, we would have legions of angry, maladjusted kids, which she just wasn't seeing.

I read this incredulous as news reports of school shootings, kids killing their parents, mothers killing their children, hazing incidents, etc. followed on the news. That is NOT to suggest low breastfeeding rates cause this angry youth, but that if this author isn't seeing these kids, it's because she is willfully choosing not to!

When the symbiotic mother-baby relationship is engaged, hormones are released each time, prolactin and oxytocin, that make babies sleep better and make mothers feel a rush of intense love. That is if the mother isn't in excruciating pain from cracked and bleeding nipples. Mothers are being told that pain in breastfeeding is normal, just as they are being led to believe pain in labor is. It is not 'normal' for your breasts to hurt while using them for the function for which they were designed! If it hurts, there is something wrong. If it is allowed to continue, it will be a miserable experience leading to probable early weaning. There may be an adjustment period, with unfamiliar and sometimes uncomfortable sensations, while mother and baby learn, but it should not be allowed to degrade into an excruciating ordeal.

Think about it...Do men need to 'prepare' their penises to ensure successful intercourse? Do they need to roughen them up with a washcloth or apply special cream? Do they need to limit their interactions to five minutes at a time until they get used to this new function? After all, there is friction and until he learns how to do this he could get blisters or something. Now, there are a hundred different things that could make sex painful, but if something hurts, he's probably not going to just continue until his penis cracks and bleeds. He's going to figure out what's wrong. What if he was told that pain in the beginning is normal, so he just keeps doing what he's doing, thinking it will go away on its own?

Feeding a baby does require coordination of partners who are both new to the relationship. It is essential that the things that are known to interfere with the relationship be avoided. It is imperative that help be sought out early if there are problems. Breastfeeding your baby is supposed to be enjoyable!

In any case, breastfeeding hormones are meant to reinforce the desire for mother to want to be around her baby, and for baby to prefer mom. This intense love is biological. When the birthing hormones are undisturbed and the nursing hormones are engaged, the result is the type of 'mother bear love' that keeps mammals from harming their offspring, makes them fiercely protective so others may not harm their offspring and triggers behaviors that make mothers want to mother. (Buckley, 2002) This foundation is very important, because when the babies reach the age of independence testing at around two, they aren't always very lovable!

The benefits of mother's milk are so numerous that entire books have been written. I suggest *Bestfeeding*, *Birthing Mother's Companion*, and *So That's What They're For!*

For now, I just want to take a common sense look at some misconceptions regarding mother's milk and artificial baby milk.

The two are often represented as 'equal' choices to mothers. This is partly because no one wants to make a mother feel guilty if she can't nurse. However, many women have problems breastfeeding not because actually can't, but because they get bad information and no support. Sometimes what they really mean is not that they can't but they won't.

Who might foster this idea of 'not making mothers feel guilty' because they make a lot of money if mothers think a substitute is just as good as human mother's milk for human babies?

The one ingredient listed in the first four in a milk substitute that isn't an allergen is sugar. Childhood obesity and diabetes have reached epidemic proportions. There is no doubt that lack of exercise and junk food contribute, but we have to acknowledge that we start the trend in infancy when we confine babies to car seats when they aren't even in the car, and assault their poor little systems with the equivalent of baby junk food.

Artificial baby milk (ABM) was made for babies whose mothers had died with no available wet nurse (other lactating mother who could feed the child).

Orphans and infants whose mothers have had their breasts removed due to cancer, or the small fraction of women who have defects of the breasts that do not allow them to nurse, need an artificial mother's milk substitute to survive.

Is it a woman's choice to bottle-feed? Of course. No one can force you to stay pregnant if you don't want to and no one can force you to use your breasts against your will. Lactation is a continuation of parturition, but it's your body, your choice. "Is it in the best interest of the child to bottle feed?" is the question.

That's what all the work you've been doing in this book comes down to. It's time to get honest about this stuff, not to make mothers 'feel' anything particular, for they can choose to feel what they want to feel. It's about the babies. It's about coming clean and getting real for the sake of the babies. As grown ups, mothers have choices, babies don't. It's up to us to make sure women have the information they need to make the best choices they can for their babies. Because we haven't been getting the truth for such a long time, the truth is going to be hard to take at first. I have faith in mothers, though. I know that once mothers can face the truth, they will do the best they can.

It isn't fair to them to enable denial and foster blame. Allowing parents to reclaim the mantle of responsibility allows them to take back their power. The art of effective parenting is on the verge of being lost as parents give their power away to 'authorities' in books. The only authority on your child is YOU. By making choices consistent with the five standards, you will be confident enough to make your own best choices as a parent.

Will parents find information on making their own best choices in the 'usual' places?

Do hospital classes and pop-culture birthing book selections give you what you need to put together the elements of a great birth?

Nope.

Those sources tell you what you want to hear because it sells. They reason it's for your own self-preservation that they can't be straight with you. It might hurt your feelings if the facts don't mesh with your beliefs. I believe parents are fed up with the results that sort of thinking leads to. I don't think it gives parents the credit they deserve for trying to do the best they can for their babies. I believe that parents who have made the effort to get this far in this book want to do the work that will get them better results than what everyone else is getting.

Those classes and those books will give you information that may seem 'balanced' in that they present all options as equal. They are lying to you, because all options aren't equal, but as long as they give the appearance of balance people will keep coming.

Independent classes are your best chance for real information not just on childbirth, but regarding breastfeeding as well.

I mentioned independent classes before. What are 'independent' classes? Most people assume that a hospital class is the only choice they have, but there are many, many choices in childbirth education.

A hospital class is a reasonable choice if it isn't a co-opted class (i.e. taught under the auspices of prominent childbirth education classes, but altered to conform to the hospital's preferences). Often you can tell what sort of class you are being offered if it is called 'prepared childbirth' instead of 'natural childbirth' and has as much (or more) of the syllabus devoted to the hospital's machines that go beep as is devoted to natural comfort techniques. Also, often the less expensive the class is, them more co-opted it has become, because it is being subsidized by drug and formula companies.

160

Leading childbirth education organizations acknowledge that childbirth education is integral to a safe, empowering birth and that leads to more confident parenting. Non-medically indicated interventions are discouraged.

However, the official stance and what parents encounter in their hospital co-opted classes are often very different. Instructors in hospitals are usually nurses who must comply with policies they have no hand in drafting. They can't discuss home birth or midwifery. They must give out formula samples, if that's the agreement the hospital arranges with the formula company. They may not be able to fully disclose the dangers of certain interventions if doctors in their hospital use those interventions routinely. Rarely does a hospital co-opted instructor have the freedom to teach per the mission of better birth adopted by nearly all of the major childbirth education associations. Often the instructor does not believe in those tenets herself. Classes may be between 4 and 6 weeks, but are often truncated to a bare minimum of classes that tell you what to expect from that particular facility.

In chat rooms and in mother's groups many mothers report that hospital classes are not helpful to them. Results seem to support that assessment, considering the high rates of epidural use and surgical births. It would seem results indicate either the comfort techniques being taught in such classes are not effective or women are not being educated about their options. Perhaps both.

The reason for this is that the classes no longer contain all of the elements that allowed mothers early on to have painless births. "Technique" has been reduced down to 'breathing.'

Hospital classes are subsidized by formula/drug companies (which are usually one and the same, i.e. Bristol-Myers, Abbott Laboratories), so they are the least expensive. However, your childbirth class is not the place where you want to try to economize. There are many options out there, so find the one that fits your learning style and has the same vision of birth that you do.

A few options are:

Mongan Method HypnoBirthing® does have all of the elements for shorter, more comfortable labor and birthing. Mickey Mongan, the originator, tries to assure that the program is not adulterated or diluted. HypnoBirthing® is a 5 week course that mainly focuses on the relaxation techniques. Complications are not discussed because most women will not encounter them, so 'why go there?' The philosophy is that our bodies know how to give birth and very often our minds just muck it up, so why complicate the process with a bunch of stuff you don't need? Keeping it simple is the plan.

Of all of the 'methods' today, this one is the most exciting in that the mothers are reporting 'fairy tale births.' Their testimonials can be found on the official website. *

Beware that you are getting the original Mongan Method HypnoBirthing®. Due to the success these mothers are having, many hospitals and others are saying they are teaching this when they are not. This is what happened to classes that became institutionalized...reducing what parents get to something nearly worthless. It's the original that is helping women birth gently, not the rip offs.

The class fee includes a book and CDs. Prices vary greatly. Practitioners who started out as childbirth educators and learned hypnosis tend to be on the low end of the scale, practitioners who started out as hypnotherapists tend to be on the high end of the scale, and those who are HypnoBirthing® practitioners only tend to be somewhere in the middle. Contact the HypnoBirthing® Institute for their preferred list of practitioners in your area.

The Association of Labor Assistants and Childbirth Educators (ALACE) is a non-profit organization that certifies childbirth educators. These classes are very balanced as far as providing factual information of all options. Deep relaxation techniques are taught.
* See 'resources' section for childbirth education websites.

Parents learn about avoiding unnecessary interventions, being informed consumers, and in some cases there is a class on complications. ALACE instructors have a great deal of freedom in what they may teach. They may be certified by other organizations besides ALACE. The classes may range from weekend 'get-away while you can still be alone' seminars, to up to 12 weeks, depending on the amount covered. Classes may be anything from just birthing information to pregnancy, birth and parenting. For parents or mothers-to-be who are "information gatherers", this is going to be the class that gives you the most for your money. Prices vary because there are so many variables in what might be offered.

The International Childbirth Education Association (ICEA) is another organization that provides professional certification programs. Like ALACE, it is an umbrella for so much more. Contact ICEA for more information.*

Bradley® Husband-Coached Childbirth classes boast a high percentage (about 80%) of natural birth success. The classes can run 8-12 weeks and are somewhat high-end in pricing for the most part.

Birthing from Within Childbirth Preparation classes are an innovative approach to childbirth education. It is an awesome resource for pregnant mothers!

As you can see from the few listed here, parents can find a childbirth class to meet any need. Restricting yourself to what 'everyone else does' will only get you what everyone else got. The numbers say that's a very sad limitation to place on yourself.

She's so lucky!

Does 'luck' play a part in what you can expect in birth? Does prayer? Synchronicity? I don't know how much any of these things might affect birth outcome. What I do know is that in birth there is a very strong cause-and-effect relationship between the choices mothers make, or allow to be made for them.

Birth is very predictable most of the time. Babies come out. How mothers feel about it, how fathers react, how caregivers interact; many of these variables are, or can be, under your control. There are just so few variables that are unknown. It is undeniable that on occasion the unpredictable occurs. Still, it is rare. Certainly, it doesn't happen as often as parents have been led to believe.

Nasty 'surprises' are only happening with such frequency in medically managed birth as it stands because it is set up that way. When more people start making choices from a place of knowledge instead of from a place of fear, this reality will be amazingly clear.

Journal Exploration:

What are your limiting beliefs about your ability to birth joyfully? Here are some common ones to help you recognize the sort of thing you might be looking for:

Birth hurts, everyone knows that!
Maybe some women can do it without drugs, but I can't even deal with a hangnail!
Some women just get lucky and have easy labors.
Why get my hopes up? Something could go wrong at any moment.
I couldn't do it last time, why would this time be different?
My body has failed me before, I should just plan on the worst.
I don't deserve a comfortable birth, it's God's will that women suffer.

You will know limiting beliefs by the finality of language such as, "always," "never," "everyone" as well as by their rigidity. Any belief that disallows new thinking or ideas is likely a limiting belief. If it has gone unchallenged up until now, it threatens your ability to create a better birth if you fail to address it. Do you have fixed beliefs about:

Doctors/Midwives:

Home birth:

Nurses:

Hospitals/Birth Centers:

Your mother's/sister's/friend's birth experience:

Your partner:

Your ability to mother (or father):

Babies:

Pregnancy, Labor, Birth:

PART THREE
Internalization

You'll see better birth when you believe it. Part three expands on the concepts of comfortable birth as a real possibility in the rite of passage that is birth.

CHAPTER 7

Birth Rite

Birth should be the most instinctual thing a woman does in her life. It is designed to be safe and effective at perpetuating the species. Certain built in mechanisms work at the instinctual and biological levels to ensure we will put our offspring above all else.

I put the work into this book to help women who are dissatisfied with their options…who are looking ahead at their probable outcome with disappointment, and already dread their expected experience. I wrote it for women who instinctively know something isn't right about birth today, but didn't have a clue what's been so wrong about it.

It's for women who want their undisturbed birthing hormones to bond them so deeply with their baby that they don't want to be apart from them. It's for women who want quick, comfortable labors without fearing they are sacrificing their baby's health or their own safety. It's for women who refuse to believe that it's

> "TRUST ONE WHO HAS GONE THROUGH IT."
> VIRGIL
> THE AENEID

'normal' for nipples to crack and bleed from using their breasts in the way nature intended. It's for women who want to spare themselves, their babies, and their families the pain and suffering they see around them in the way of rising rates of postpartum depression. It's for women who know this mothering gig is hard enough without manufactured obstacles to overcome.

It's also for those women who are past childbearing, who did the best they could with what they had, and may feel cheated with what they got, who want better for their sisters, friends and daughters.

The essential elements known to result in safe childbearing are referred to repeatedly, as is the concept of evidence-based care.

These are ideals resulting in safer mothers and healthier babies. By knowing what produces optimal outcomes, you can strive for your own best outcome possible in your individual circumstance. If we want mothers and babies, thus society, to reach our highest potential, we need to strip away the illusions that dilute or contaminate our perception of empowered, safe birth.

In order to discover your personal best, you must be completely honest with yourself. No one has to be privy to any of internal exploration you may include in your journal, so even painful or 'politically incorrect' thoughts can be explored. It's time to ask yourself if the filter through which you view your pregnancy and birth is causing you to dismiss options as unobtainable, when the reality may be that they are as available to you as anyone else.

So often options are invisible to us, even when they are well within reach. We trap ourselves with our own limited thinking. The universe is so much more generous with us than we are to ourselves!

By being honest about what doesn't create a safe, dignified and empowering birth, we can identify and implement what does.

Taking ownership of the parts of pregnancy and birth you can control allows you to accept what you can't. By acknowledging your role in the creation of your birth experience, it's possible that you can improve your outcome.

If you are a healthy woman and you still haven't become a partner in your care after reading this far, there must be factors you are not acknowledging that drive your behavior, such as unconscious fear. If you are still consenting to routine prenatal technologies, if you haven't interviewed a midwife, if you haven't made an effort to learn about normal pregnancy and birth by reading any of the suggested reading in the appendix, you may ask yourself, 'why?' Why would you accept less than what you deserve?

You have to be honest with yourself if you really want a shorter, more comfortable labor with fewer complications than the national average. If you really want optimal physical and emotional health you need to make the choices we know contribute to those outcomes. These are not the same choices that are considered the 'norm' in our society right now. Unfortunately, that requires that additional effort be put forth to come up with your plan for your best birth.

Maybe there are no midwives in your area. Your choices will be different than a mother in Oregon where midwives are plentiful. You may have to look outside your geographical area for a birth center. Maybe you have no transportation, so you have to work with what you have locally, whether it's acceptable or not. You still have options. You just have to be more creative in finding them!

My point here is we always have choices—some easy, some not. It's up to us to decide what's important to us and make decisions that support what matters. We can't do that until we are honest with ourselves about what is truly important to us in our individual circumstance, and then acknowledge that we do have the power to get it.

In order to do this, you must examine and challenge every belief and position you hold in regard to pregnancy, birth, and early parenting. When we discuss the facts of what makes babies safe, healthy and well adjusted, you must be willing to honestly assess your beliefs, patterns and positions against those facts. When it comes to pregnancy, birth and parenting, you can't afford the luxury of denial. Your baby's life and future depends on you taking responsibility for that which you are responsible.

As humans, we have a self-protective 'perceptual defense.' It protects us from those things our inner self might find sort of scary. This is a wonderful gift of our wise self when it protects us from trauma. However, it could be keeping you from seeing things you simply do not want to be true. It may be causing you to dismiss your mother's intuition on a daily basis, keeping you from seeing warning signs in your caregiver's behavior or allowing you to continue behaviors you know are harmful to you or your baby.

Your subconscious mind, the seat of your mother's intuition, knows if you are not making the best choices for yourself and your baby, even if your consciousness is blocking the messages. This is where guilt and defensiveness originate. If you are blocking out the very information proven to result in what you say you want for your baby, it is unrealistic to think you will actually get it. This may be evident in conflicting words and actions. For instance, if you take the advice of this book and seek out an independent childbirth educator, but ridicule everything about it and refuse to practice techniques. Paying the fee is not the part that improves outcomes. You have to do the work. They way you approach the practice is the way you are really seeing the event.

Think of it like this: Say you wanted to make cookies and you had a great recipe. You get the recipe out and read it. Do you have cookies? No? Ok, you take out all the ingredients and set them out. Do you have cookies? What if you have most of the ingredients, but have to go to the store to find a few. You buy those, bring them home and put them with the other gathered ingredients. Cookies? Of course not. Having the raw materials and spending the money means nothing if you don't follow the directions and actually do the work of putting it all together. You need to make the necessary changes to get a better birth. Sometimes that means shifting our perceptions and expectations, which shape your outcome. We see what we want to see, sometimes with contradictory evidence staring us right in the face.

Remember the elements for safe childbearing? These have been determined, and are backed by decades of science. In the appendix you will find entire books supplying the science of what makes birth safe. Has the evidence caused you to explore your options more fully?

Years ago, two Harvard researchers won a Nobel prize for their experiment on two groups of kittens fitted with special goggles. One group was raised able to see only horizontal lines. The other group was raised seeing only vertical lines. Once grown, it was discovered the group raised in the horizontal environment didn't recognize vertical lines in a maze, and those raised in the vertical world couldn't see horizontal lines. When the brains of these animals were examined, the researches found that there were no neural connections between the neurons responsible for recognizing vertical and horizontal lines in the respective groups. The kittens raised to believe the world is vertical simply could not see any other possibility. Likewise, those raised in a horizontal 'world' could not conceive of a vertical world, not because of their psychology, but because of their physical neurological structure. (Myers, 2003)

While this study has implications reaching into the reality of how we birth and parent our babies and how their brains develop, I use it here to point out that they did not see what was clearly before them because they had no experience of a different reality. They didn't see what they didn't expect to see.

People come to childbirth classes with dread over what they will see. Women expect to see needles and cutting, men fear they will react in an 'unmanly' way to 'all that blood'. Their conception of birth includes machines, a room full of masked strangers, being confined to bed in a hospital gown open down the back, drugs, wires and tubes. Even if it's dreaded (for some wisdom deep down inside understands that this all screams 'danger') it is expected. Parents simply expect nothing else and so have a hard time picturing anything else when I try to explain that birth...normal, natural, healthy birth, which about 85-90% should be...includes NONE of these things. Because they have not been brought up to envision strong women, birthing comfortably in the nest they have create at home, with candles, their own tub, their own food, freedom of movement with those they love around them as 'normal,' the picture is a difficult one for them to form. In fact, even after trying to 'draw' this brain picture for them, some people will say 'Well sure, but who wants all that mess in their house? At the hospital they clean up all the blood!" Natural birth is very neat and usually quite clean. More than two cups of blood is a hemorrhage, which is not usual. Babies are born in a tide of clean, sterile water. If healthy tissue isn't cut, it's really not all that messy, just wet. But they shake their heads, unable to see safe birth as wonderful birth because they've been conditioned to see safe and wonderful in direct opposition.

Those of us who have seen, with our own eyes, what the evidence confirms, safe, comfortable, empowering, gentle birth, want you to see it too! Fortunately, you don't have to grow new neural connections. You just have to decide to see it.

Have you surrounded yourself with images, stories and pictures of empowered pregnancy and blissful birth? What are you conditioning your mind—and by extension your body—to accept? To expect? Are you relying on tests that in healthy women are inaccurate or useless at the expense of your intuition, your body wisdom? Your wise body knew how to create a human being from two single cells. Every day it builds these cells, organs, tissues. Amazingly, it will know when the work is done and the baby should be born, and even more amazingly, it will then know to produce the perfect food that only you can make for your baby. All of this happens without a conscious thought from you. All of it happens whether you have the tests or don't. It is happening for women with midwives, and women alone in the rainforest. Why should you be so fearful that the ubiquitous 'something' might go wrong when billions and billions of times, over thousands and thousands of years, the process worked just as it's supposed to? Yes, sometimes things happen that might have been prevented, but the scales have tipped so that now more problems are created than encountered. Vigilance and monitoring are in proportion to the risk and are appropriate, but interventions inappropriate to individual circumstance have become the norm and are creating more problems than they are solving.

Changing our point of reference again illustrates this point. A multitude of things CAN go wrong with any system in the body, but seldom actually DO. Take the heart/circulatory system, for example. Heart disease is the leading cause of death in the US. 873 per 100,000 die of heart disease (CDC). (Remember, natural birth is between 6 and 14 per 100,000 in the US, depending on the population.) Some people have arteries on the verge of clogging. Some have heart defects they are unaware of. Some people have damage they don't know about. Something could go wrong at any minute and immediately available surgery can undoubtedly save lives.

Using the logic of obstetrics, all health clubs should be in hospital and all fitness trainers should be cardiac surgeons. Any independent health club with 'lay' trainers would be 'practicing medicine without a license,' subject to prosecution. It's for your own good.

In fact, in order to know if a problem is developing, close monitoring and 'management' is required. We will need to place straps on the muscles to measure the intensity of the workout. Of course, it will be restrictive, but we need to know how hard the muscles are working to know if the heart can take it. We'll need to monitor heart rate, blood pressure, fluid output. We'll need to give an IV because with sweat excreted, you could dehydrate, and of course, we simply can't take the risk of letting you drink anything lest you need emergency surgery.

Maybe all activity that increases heart rate should be monitored. How about sex? Again, blood pressure, heart rate, IV, speed and adequacy of penile erectile performance. Bright lights and strangers assessing a man every 15 minutes or so might be a bit distracting, but medically speaking, his heart is a time bomb. We don't want men's hearts to get to the point of stress. I'm sure they would be relieved to know that if they can't get it up or keep it up, or if it looks like his body is working too hard, we can always surgically remove the sperm so that his failure doesn't damage his reproductive system.

There was a booklet out years ago called *Natural Love* by Janet Isaacs Ashford that detailed such a scenario to illustrate the parallels to birthing.

For, as ridiculous as the above sounds, it does make very clear how current birth management disrupts the process. All of the same hormones involved in sex, as well as the same organs, are involved in birth. What would make intercourse difficult or impossible? The same things disrupt the balance of birth and make it dangerous.

It's not too late to maximize your positive potential if you are honest without yourself about what needs fixing before this baby comes. It means removing the filters that convince you that the current system is just peachy, when in reality it has you on the fast track to an unnecessary surgery. It means recognizing inappropriately applied technology, as well as the emotional drain of a fear-based paradigm.

Denial allows this birth machine to keep on damaging women's lives. We all must be willing to consider our place in the system we have and own it. Being willing and able to identify and acknowledge negative attitudes, ideas or behaviors is essential in order to change them. The hard part is that on some level, the level denying what you don't want to hear which operates under a perceptual defense mechanism, you perceive these attitudes to be 'normal' responses. You may even see them as positive.

How do you know for sure which each is? Judge by results and ask yourself if the facts support the belief.

Acknowledgment means little, however, if it is not followed by commitment to change. If you want a better experience, you must make decisions that support the experience you seek. If you find yourself thinking 'yeah, but...,' you have to change that thinking. There are a lot of things in life you can put off until later, but better birth isn't one of them. Your baby is growing closer to being in your arms every single day. If you don't face your shadows before he or she is ready to make an entrance, you won't get a chance later. You can't 'take back' a birth and you don't get a dress rehearsal. You are preparing for the real deal. Remember, how you train for the game is how you play the game. The brain chemistry alterations inherent in natural birth are for keeps and they can't be made to happen at any other time. The health benefits of feeding your baby its birth right of mother's milk are life-long.

These are nature's gifts to you to make your first days as easy as possible. Thus, they happen naturally in natural birth. The are often absent in a disrupted birth. The cumulative effect of choices you make from this moment through the next several years shape the kind of person your child will be. There is no job more important.

"Yeah, but..." clearly reveals you are not accepting this absolute truth. It indicates you are making excuses for not holding yourself to the highest standard on behalf of your baby. You are settling for with less than what you and your baby deserve.

People want reinforcement and validation for what they already think, right or wrong. They intentionally seek out the people, information and support for conclusions already reached, regardless of if those conclusions rest on a factual foundation. They want to hear what makes them feel good about choices they've made, good or bad. We all have this propensity. It's called 'confirmation bias.' Mother's have been blamed for everything from bedwetting children to ax murdering adults, so the tendency is to tenaciously defend any choices mothers make to over compensate for decades of unfairness. This is not helping to create a better reality. The truth lies in the middle. Mothers are not to blame for everything wrong in the world...but they have the power to make so much right.

Sadly, I know there will be some women who will be resistant to this idea. We have legions of mothers walking wounded. The truth comes too late for them and that's painful. I wish there was a way to help those hurting moms while helping moms-to-be.

There will be women who simply will choose to ignore all of this good advice. That's fine, too. Keep telling yourself you can't have a better birth and you'll be right. You make yourself right by your actions. If you'd rather make decisions based on beliefs with no basis in fact, rather than be empowered, safe and comfortable at your birth, it is your choice to make.

Normal and natural aren't as hard to access as some would have you believe, though. Mothers with strong intuition have bravely maintained the natural that should be 'normal' on the outskirts. That is how we even have the data to compare what we have with what we've lost…or nearly lost. Follow the examples of these mothers and change for the better will happen — one mother-baby at a time. Birth is a defining moment in a woman's life.

It can be very threatening to acknowledge a problem that is so big and complex. I'm fully aware that change is never easy and that as mothers reclaim ownership over their part of the problem there will be resistance from everyone that prefers things just the way they are. There are people with quite a financial stake in the current system, from pharmaceutical/formula companies to obstetricians as well as those too afraid to face their own fears.

"The hand that rocks the cradle rules the world" may be cliché, but it is reality. When mothers take back birth, when more and more mothers begin to tell their joyful stories, transformation is inevitable. When mothers realize what they've been missing, they will be a force to reckon with.

My wish for women is comfortable, safe birth. My wish for babies is health and stability. My wish for dads is a bonded, happy family. My wish for doctors is freedom from fear of litigation. My wish for midwives the freedom to practice their passion.

I know everyone isn't ready, willing and able to break through the system that keeps us in a self-destruct mode, but some people are more than ready. This is for those who know there are no accidents, accepting ownership for the experience they are creating for themselves. It's for the parents willing to commit to be genuinely honest with themselves. Be willing to ask yourself the hard questions and face your own truth with no lies, no excuses...no telling yourself what you want to be, instead of what is.

Admit to yourself if—

--you are scared of birth
--you feel you don't deserve a wonderful birth
--you feel powerless in your pregnancy --you are allowing other people to make your birthing decisions
--you are just maintaining, day by day, with no positive expectations for your baby's birth
--you are not requiring the best of yourself for your baby
--you are self-destructive in ways that could affect your baby
--you are breaking promises to yourself or your partner
--you are breaking promises to your baby

A great deal of the solution is defining the problem. Once you have the courage to admit that fear or belief may be in the way of seeing the truth about the most common aspects of obstetrically managed birth you will be unable to accept the myths leading to the frustration so prevalent in mothers and children today.

The way we currently view birth did not happen overnight or by accident and it won't change without conscious intent. We need to stop making excuses for the inexcusable. You must accept responsibility for just this one thing and create something better for yourself if you want better...instead of 'good enough.'

Admitting to being scared or confused about this powerful, mysterious thing called birth is not weakness. It is the first step to empowerment. Being honest with ourselves allows us to stop accepting so little for ourselves and start making changes. You'll be a better mother for it because you'll be a better person. You have to want it for yourself and for your baby.

It's not about anyone else's expectations for your birth. It's about you knowing you, your baby and your family deserve the best.

Give yourself permission to deal with any distorted beliefs, thoughts or feelings about birth. Our culture has heaped a whole lot of nonsense on mothers...baggage that we have to deal with. Allow yourself to take it one step at a time. Be gentle with yourself.

You are the parent you are because of your life experiences. You have incorporated these experiences, events and ideas and they impact every pregnancy, birthing and parenting decision you make. Accepting that some of these experiences are different than how they may have appeared through our personal filter is imperative. Allow this distortion to be revealed by educating yourself on what is really natural and normal in birth. Know what is actually possible through better decision-making. You will stand a much greater chance of having the 'fairy tale birth' other women only dream about.

Journal Exploration:

What are your conscious parenting decisions? For example:

I will respect my baby's dignity, treating him or her with kindness and patience.
I will be the best parent I can be, learning what I don't already know.
I will not harm or allow others to harm my baby, as protective as a mother bear.

These are the commitments that guide your behavior all of the time. These are your convictions. These are the things you will not compromise. You may be very proud that you are already experiencing motherhood with your head, heart and hands. Or, you may be disappointed in yourself if you are failing to live up to your ideal. How will you deal with set backs and how much effort are you willing to put forth for the sake of your baby?

MY COMMITMENTS:

CHAPTER 8
Intentions and Expectations

It's not what we say that matters, it's what we do. It is not our intentions that create change, but our actions.

This chapter points out that intent without action means nothing in pregnancy and birth. Very often today, a 'successful' birth is judged by whether a mother has a live, healthy baby in her arms. Of course, we all agree. What seems to have been lost is that it is what we should expect, since the overwhelming majority of time, that is the way nature works. It has become the hallmark of a 'good birth' intentionally…because it is justification for all of the sacrifices mothers are needlessly required to make. Iatrogenic (doctor caused) and nosocomial (hospital caused) complications are considered acceptable because, of course, all that matters is a healthy mother and baby. This idea makes the parent feel ungrateful for expecting more, even though the mother's life that will never, ever really 'be the same'.

I know of no other area of medicine (or any other profession) where someone is thanked for creating a problem…even if they can fix it.

What if…

You went to the doctor complaining of chest pain…not bad pain, but bothersome. To rule out a heart problem, the caregiver listens to your heart. He scowls, then excuses himself to make a phone call. He comes back in and tells you that you need to be admitted to the hospital for a test that requires the use of a drug. The drug has a low risk of serious complications, which is why you must be in the hospital, but he feels confident in taking that risk.

You go, and within minutes of having the drug administered, you have a heart attack. You are rushed into emergency open-heart surgery. Complications arise, but they are dealt with. You nearly bleed to death, but with blood replacement you recover.

The repair doesn't go well, which may mean you will need further surgery later...maybe even a heart transplant. You definitely will need to change your previously active lifestyle.

Later, you discover the call your care provider placed was to an HMO lawyer who advised him not to let you walk out the door, just in case the routine examination missed a serious problem. You also learn that there were less dangerous ways, though perhaps more expensive than the drug, or perhaps not current 'standard of care' to determine if there could be a minor problem. And as it turns out, all you really had was a pulled muscle. All you have been through was avoidable, but "As long as everyone's ok now...that's all that matters"...right?

A comment like that, to a mother who has suffered unnecessarily, when she would have-or could have-had the result of a live, healthy baby without such sacrifice, disregards her feelings of loss.

Parents should be expecting more!

When women discuss their upcoming births, they say, "I'm going to try to have a natural birth, but..." The statement is rift with subconscious communicators.

To say one will 'try', instead of calmly stating that they will be having a natural birth, implies a.) there is no belief that it can or will be accomplished and b.) the effort factor can be very low because there is no commitment. The 'but' at the end of the statement further tells us to negate everything that came before it. So, forget the first half of the sentence and listen to the last half, for that's where the real beliefs are.

Up until now, most of what readers have been asked to do throughout this book is internal. Even if this is as far as you go, if

184

you've done the work, you can't help but have new and exciting ideas about pregnancy, birth and parenting.

If, however, it's a better birth you want, you will need to act on your newfound perspective. I believe most mothers intend to make the safest choices for their babies. The ones who intend, but act contrary to all evidence of safety, have contributed to the current birth statistics that have been outlined here. Few set out to be an unnecessary cesarean, a figure in the outrageously high US mortality rate or a victim of any one of the preventable postpartum problem figures. They just intended to 'try' to give birth the way most of their friends 'tried' to give birth. If you want a great birth, you have to plan the way mothers who have had great births planned.

To create the birth you want, your behaviors must constructively reflect the better birth you want to create. Better choices backed by actions produce results. Intention without action is just wishful thinking, and the odds are against your wishes coming true if you are a healthy woman being obstetrically managed.

By now, if you've been doing the work, you will have identified changes that could be made in your pregnancy, birth and parenting plan that would improve your experience. Have you made those changes? Are you thinking about it? Have you dismissed them?

Take the following test to see where you stand:

	Yes	No
1. Do you regularly watch crisis oriented birthing programs?	___	___
2. Do you eat fast food more often than fresh food?	___	___
3. Are you still seeing a caregiver that keeps you waiting for two hours at every appointment?	___	___

Yes   No

4. On the internet, you find a website where women
   post their birth stories. Do you dismiss the stories
   of painless, orgasmic 2-hour labors as unattainable,
   as you dish with friends who tell you
   how it really is?   ___   ___

5. Has your due date 'changed' because your ultrasound
says so? (How many times has your
conception date changed?)   ___   ___

6. Do you spend more time watching TV
than reading about better birth or taking classes?   ___   ___

7. Are the only books on your shelf the ones
your doctor 'allows'?   ___   ___

8. Do you spend more time online than on
your relationship with your baby's father?   ___   ___

9. When you envision your birth,
are you surrounded by masked strangers?   ___   ___

10. Are you suspicious of mothers who seem blissful?   ___   ___

11. Do you feel that you'll never have a wonderful birth
because...(fill in the blank with any prenatal test scare)   ___   ___

12. Are you afraid birth will be the most excruciating
event you'll ever experience?   ___   ___

13. Are your days full of worry that 'something'
will go wrong?   ___   ___

14. Do you feel ill equipped to be a mother?   ___   ___

15. Are you more concerned about appearances
of competence than actually learning competency?
(i.e. taking the childbirth class, but not doing the work) ___ ___

16. Do you find yourself afraid to ask questions
of your caregiver?   ___ ___

17. Do you find yourself saying 'yes' to prenatal tests,
interventions or plans you don't want and for which
you question the need?   ___ ___

If you said 'yes' to any of these you have plenty of company…women who had exactly the kind of birth they didn't want, but didn't do a thing except wish for a different outcome. If you said 'yes' to less than half of these questions, you need to decide on at least 10 new actions if you want to change the course of your pregnancy outcome.

If you said yes to more than half, you need to rethink everything to have a better birth.

Journal Exploration:

How healthy are your relationships with those persons involved in your pregnancy and birth?

Do you feel your partner controls your birthing choices?

Is your relationship with your caregiver more like parent/child than equality between adults?

Do you and your partner, parents and friends argue over your safe & gentle birth choices?

Do you find yourself apologizing to your care provider for what should be reasonable expectations & requests?

Do you feel that during your pregnancy you have made more concessions and compromises than anyone else?

Do you frequently make excuses for your partner & care provider when discussing their involvement in the direction your birth is heading?

Do you feel your emotional needs are either not being met or are being played upon?

Do you feel that choices made by others regarding your pregnancy and birth are-or may be-cheating you out of enjoying your experience?

Do your pregnancy/birth discussions with your partner (your care provider, your family, your friends) leave you frustrated, exhausted or afraid?

Do you feel your wants and needs are not a priority to your caregiver or partner?

Do you have ideas about how you want your pregnancy and birth to be that you don't share with your partner or care provider?

Do you feel devalued?

Do you secretly believe other people are leading you to a less than desirable birth experience?

Do you see negative patterns to your relationships with those in your planned birth party?

Do you feel afraid to be vulnerable in any of your birthing relationships?

Do you feel you are the only one willing to work for better birth?

Do you feel emotionally detached from those who will be a part of this most emotional event, including your baby?

Do you feel you've had to give up dreams, or expectations, of a better birth to keep peace in your relationship with your partner, care provider, family or friends?

Are you just coasting along, not making waves, hoping for a decent birth?

Are you seeing your care provider just because you started out there, or because someone you know did, rather than finding someone you really like or are comfortable with?

You've bought this book and come this far, so part of you must want a great birth. What is holding you back from making it a reality? Translating your new insights and awareness into meaningful action is the only way to get what you want.

Commit to measuring your progress by results, not intent. It's natural tend to make excuses. Most people do it. It's natural to avoid change. Most people don't like it.

"SO OFTEN WOMEN WILL TRY TO CHANGE THEIR CAREGIVER WITH EVERY VISIT...INSTEAD OF CHANGING CAREGIVERS."
KIM WILDNER

It's not unusual to defer responsibility, either. Our society seems to embrace the victim mentality and the blamers, illustrated by our astronomical malpractice rates and ridiculous lawsuits. It is not ok, just typical. In this instance 'not my job, not my fault' is not an option. You grow this baby, you birth this baby, you need to raise this baby. You and your baby are your only priority.

I'm not interested in helping you make a birth wish list. Plenty of people make a 'birth plan' that includes avoiding lots of stuff they may actually need because the foundation of a healthy pregnancy through optimal nutrition is missing. New insights into the nature of birth mean nothing if it stops there.

When mothers get fed up, when they stand up and yell "We're mad as hell and we're not taking it anymore!"...only then will birth on the whole improve. It starts with you. Do you and your baby deserve better? Make it happen.

There are no do-overs, if this is your first baby, that means all you have are other people's results to assess where the actions you have in common will probably lead. I have included relevant data and resources throughout the book for you to follow up on so you may asses your own situation. I don't know what choices are best for you, but I want to help you figure out what choices are best. Self-evaluation is the only evaluation that matters. The only way to determine where you are and where you're going is to assess feelings and facts. Neither has a thing to do with 'intending' to do anything. A healthy pregnancy, peaceful pregnancy and good birth require investment. Good parenting requires investment of self.

Your midwife doesn't care that you intend to stop smoking if you keep on smoking. Your body and your baby don't care what your intentions are. If you keep smoking, your body reacts to your actions, not your intentions. Your baby reacts to your actions, not your intentions. Your midwife must react to your actions.

This commitment means not making excuses for, or taking excuses from, your caregiver or your partner either. If you decided you will expect better treatment from other people, measure that treatment by their actions, not their words.

For your provider to tell you she has every intention of 'letting' you have a natural birth means nothing if she's treating you like a sick person and talking about inducing you based on irrelevant findings from a routine ultrasound. Are you going to spend your entire pregnancy letting machines and tests tell you how you feel? Dismissing your wise body and built-in mother's intuition because a test, known to be highly unreliable, says something different?

Start requesting documentation of safety and efficacy before consenting to any test or intervention. A good doctor will welcome this. It's called informed consent and it protects them as well as you. A bad doctor will pay lip service, maybe even treating you condescendingly or lying. Until we sort out the good from the bad, unfortunately, that means checking and double-checking. Again, good and trustworthy caregivers will not take offense at this.

Decline testing for the sake of testing. Decline interventions that don't benefit you. Yes, this means doing your homework. You will be paving the way for the women behind you, perhaps providing healing for some of the women before.

Eventually, outcomes improve and more women are telling wonderful stories instead of sad ones.

Change caregivers if your current one is threatened by you being a partner in your own pregnancy decisions. If you are told you have a condition for which you need a particular test, intervention or cesarean, look up the condition. Ask to see the evidence indicating you have it. Know what 'normal' is for you.

If your doctor starts talking surgery at 30 weeks because your baby is breech and he says there no way to turn a breech or deliver breech safely, look it up. If a doctor lies to you, even once, it's NOT OK. Before 34-36 weeks it means absolutely nothing to you if your baby is butt first. You still have time to find a new care provider. It doesn't matter if you are two weeks away from birthing or actually in labor. You don't have to put up with unacceptable treatment from anyone privileged enough to be allowed at your baby's entrance into this world!

You can ignore the truth, but that won't change it. When people show you who they are, believe them. The number one job of a mother is to protect her baby from harm. You accepted that job the instant you decided to be pregnant.

It's a gift to be entrusted with a tiny new life to love and care for. It's an honor. Becoming a parent with no regrets means standing up for what you know in your heart is right for you and your child and not making excuses.

We plan every detail of our weddings, from the guest list to the menu. We arrange everything months in advance, we comparison shop. We map out a course for college. We plan a schedule that will advance us toward a goal and we make sacrifices along the way. We sometimes have to get creative in ways to pay for it.

Birth requires the same dedication, the same love. We cannot put off thinking about it until the last minute, expecting someone else to take care of everything. Well, we can, and we have...it's what has created the mess we have now.

No one loves your baby more than you. It's not someone else's job to make everything all right. It's an impossible expectation to think someone else can put your baby's needs before their own. Heck, there are a lot of parents that aren't willing to do that, who expects a stranger to?

How much time have you got left in this pregnancy? You get one chance at this first face-to-face meeting with the one you'll love beyond reason until the day you die. Be committed to a better birth, do what it takes to create it and you will have the most rewarding experience possible.

A month from now, you might have read all the books listed in the appendix and your entire birthing paradigm may have shifted, but if you don't do anything with your new-found knowledge, it doesn't mean a thing. Better birth doesn't happen by osmosis.

If you know the elements of a better birth, yet you do nothing about it, you don't get a better birth. If you know what makes birth into a scary, dangerous, medical event and you allow those elements to prevail in your care, you get the scary, dangerous, medical event.

You can tell yourself, "well, I know all this to be true, and I really want to have a home birth, but I'll do it next time" know that is highly unlikely to happen. You have a 1 in 3 chance of ending up with surgery, which affects future pregnancy expectations. Even if you don't end up with unnecessary surgery, surrounding yourself with a crisis orientation while you are in the highly suggestible state that is birth will reinforce the idea of 'birth = crisis.' A multitude of iatrogenic or nosocomial complications will give substance to every subconscious fear you have about birth. Home birthing moms hear stories constantly that begin with "I could never have had my baby at home because..." with some awful account of an event in which birth was messed up by something a doctor or other staff did.

The difference between healthy mothers and babies having nightmarish births and those who have the dreamy version hinges on what they do. Fairy-tale birth mothers don't just think about how to create better birth, they make it happen. They actively avoid what they don't want and they work towards what they do want. They approach motherhood the same way. If one of the rare complications occurs that justifies an assortment of interventions that they'd rather avoid, they accept the turn their birthing takes because they know they've encountered a situation, not created it.

Letting someone else have control over your pregnancy and birth does ensure there is no pressure to be accountable for results. Some people prefer the option of blaming others. I would think doctors would discourage this dependency instead of fostering it, but that doesn't seem to be so.

Thus far we've explored what the overall problem with current standard of care is, how it could affect your birth and what role your subconscious core beliefs play in what reality you create. You know that knowing about better options, combined with doing better, means having a better birth.

To get healthy results instead of unhealthy ones, do you need to make some changes? Do you want step-by-step instructions on what to do with what you are discovering? We'll get to how to prioritize your time and energy.

As you create the reality that is your birth, that is your experience as a new parent, through your own actions, the choices will be yours. Your parenting choices will not be the same as mine or anyone else's. We all know what's important to us. Do we act on it? Or do we react…to circumstances we didn't intend, but did nothing to prevent?

Do something different, something important to improve your birth and your life as a new mother.

194

You can help change the world, one baby at a time, if you start to do different things than 'everyone else' does.

Notice 'I wanted to but...' or 'I wish I could _____ but...' statements. These are excuses if the 'but' isn't followed by an actual uncontrollable variable. If you want something bad enough, there is almost always a way to make it happen. The very rare instance of unexpected, uncontrolled outcomes has been blown out of proportion to justify a system that cannot be justified with the facts. There is no doubt that once in a great while bad stuff happens to good people. For now, know that the vast majority can find a way to create birth the experience they want or to breastfeed. What if other natural physiological functions were approached with the mindset that a very small possibility of misfortune is an excuse to medically manage the function? It's a known fact that people die in choking deaths, so should all people get their nutrition from an IV and never eat again to eliminated the remote possibility of choking?

Sometimes just seeing that meaningful change is contingent on being skeptical of 'the way things are' helps us to begin 'examining everything we have been told and rejecting what insults our soul.' Question everything you think you know about birth.

Question how and where you focus your attention and spend your time. What does 'self-talk' sound like? How do you interact with those to be involved in the single most significant event in your life? This is a huge opportunity to contribute positively to your world, and all you have to do is take back what is already yours.

Have you familiarized yourself with the concept of comfortable birth without drugs? Do you know how to achieve it? If not, take a Mongan Method HypnoBirthing® class. Have you made out a birth plan of your preferences and discussed it with your caregiver? Do you know what his or her preferences are? Are they evidence-based? Do they match with your preferences? Are they conducive to gentle birth? If not, have you sought out other providers? Why or why not?

Are you healing from a past birth experience? Did you feel powerless? Vulnerable? Abused? Violated? Wounded, physically and emotionally? Did your experience leave you with precious little reserves to be the mother you wanted to be? Have you been told you should just feel lucky anyway? Basically having your need to grieve discounted as trivial? Have you been manipulated so that you feel guilty for being angry, for even allowing your strong mother's intuition to suggest that it's all wrong?

Pushing down those painful feelings only means they will resurface later. You don't deserve to feel bad now and you don't need to feel it again later, maybe in the form of depression or anger, maybe at a subsequent birth. Maybe even misdirected at your baby.

Use any pain that surfaces to get you moving toward a gentle birth this time. Consciously creating a better birth can be a healing force. A gentle, natural, safe birth can empower a woman. Empowered women change the world. Allow your pain to be motivation to make birth better, safer, for yourself and for your daughters after you. After your birth, we can be one step deeper into what already isn't working for anyone, or we can be one step closer to healthy, strong moms and healthy, peaceful babies.

Some people are born early adopters. They question everything. They thrive on being different. They are unwilling to settle for 'because I said so.' They refuse to settle for 'good enough.' If you are one of those people, you will embrace what you have learned here and be a positive force in improving birth. Possibly angry at first that you never knew the truth about birth today and no one ever suggested you ask.

Some, on the other hand, don't work without a constant safety net. They settle for what feels wrong because it feels safer than not having a guarantee that they'll get what they want, even if it's a false sense of security. Those of you who prefer illusionary comfort zones to grounded stability in the 'unknown' or the 'different' may have a harder time embracing better birth, because it's uncommonly found around you. You must seek out the components and put them together yourself. It's still attainable…you'll just need to stretch way beyond what you have ever done before. You will be transformed if you take on the challenge for the sake of your baby.

It may feel as if your peace of mind or relationships will be put at risk if you step outside the box. You may feel tension between wanting to maintain the false security of 'sameness' and the excitement of actually getting a fabulous birth. The very act of admitting you want a better birth is too big to contemplate.

Familiar ideas, even if they are false assumptions, are predictable, like a 'frenemy' you know you should dump but don't. Our medicalized vision of birth makes one wonder, 'Better birth sounds great, but what if it's not real? How bad can it get?' In childbearing, obviously the stakes are high. How do you know which vision of birth is real? Which is safe? Test the validity of both. Just because you see birth through culturally imposed blinders doesn't mean what you see is real. Test both visions against facts, data, and evidence. You will see that you have nothing to lose by checking out what I have been saying. In the years since I have been a childbirth professional, birth has only gotten more dangerous. United States statistics have only worsened. Mothers have only become more unhappy. Babies have grown to very disturbed adolescents. I'd like to say it can't get worse, but it can, and it is. However, the good news is that if you make choices based on what we know to be the elements of safe childbearing, if you refute the lies that have been foisted upon us, if you take the less traveled, unfamiliar path, it can't be worse than what we have now.

Birth related fear comes in many flavors. Maslow's Hierarchy of Needs puts fear of rejection as a high priority for humans. As mothers, a fear of death or pain ranks right up there in the first three contenders. Results would suggest they aren't #1 or #2, for if we feared death the most, women would not choose to birth in the hospital with a conventional obstetrician…one place she will most assuredly feel pain and is most at risk because of it. If the number one fear was pain, coupled with baby's safety, women would seek out alternatives in such numbers that we practitioners would be teaching several full classes every single day, midwives would be swamped and obstetrical care would be forced to transform.

Fear of rejection, of being odd-man-out or being seen as weird, keeps us doing things that are harmful to us, just because 'everyone else does it.' What if you face your birthing fears? What if you make choices in your pregnancy and parenting career that your friends don't understand? What if you are willing to believe in painless birth? What if you are willing to validate the safety of home birth, if it is indeed safe for your circumstance? What if you do make a different choice and something goes wrong?

'Something'...countless 'somethings' go wrong everyday in hospitals. No one suggests that these women 'failed.' Why are the standards different for women willing to make choices based on fact instead of fear? This double standard makes women feel as if they are putting themselves out on a limb, even though the opposite is true. Are you sticking with a false sense of security at the expense of your hopes and dreams?

Is an unwillingness to put energy into constructive action towards better birth justified? OR is it unreasonable fear paralyzing your actions? Allow yourself to feel the fear—and do it anyway. Let unfounded fears be someone else's concern. You have another life to consider. You don't have the privilege of hiding behind fear.

However seemingly illogical your mind may want to make the facts of gentle birth, they are the facts. Gauge success by the birth data.

You deserve to feel pride and strength in your accomplishment of growing a human being and bringing him or her into the world. Make the effort, be persistent, and take back your birth. Better birth won't happen to you by accident. It will happen only because you make it happen. If you do, there will be no regrets, no shame.

Work from where you are currently in your pregnancy with a fresh perspective. If regrets or shame have plagued you from a previous birth experience, work to release or reframe those experiences so that you can be present in the now for this baby.

You cannot have an unnecessarily traumatic birth if you haven't made choices that support unnecessary trauma. Your choices will support a traumatic birth or a better birth. You decide.

Unavoidable trauma is a rare occurrence. Expect normal, accept the unexpected. Manage what you are presented with. The more we take charge of creating better birth, the easier it will be to see that what we expect from birth now has been created and is not the birth experience Nature wished for us.

Journal Exploration:

The current birth environment is rift with abdication of responsibility and blame. In this exercise, identify those situations that created anger, resentment or frustration in a past birth or your current pregnancy. Once the origin of the trauma is identified, love yourself and your baby enough to let it go. By forgiving yourself and others, you can empower yourself in your current pregnancy instead of letting past events control this outcome.

Start by looking for 'blaming' statements in your own situation. These may be similar to the earlier ones in bold. For doctors and other caregivers, this type of statement might include, "The client insisted."
Realize that others in these situations may have chosen different problem solving techniques and achieved different outcome. All of the sample statements required compliance on the part of another.

Write down as many possible options for each situation as you can. Understand that you may have knowledge now you may not have had at the time of the event.

Now, forgive yourself and the other party so you can release negative emotion. You might do this by writing a letter and then burning it. If it's safe to do so, you may wish to converse with the other person in a constructive way to ensure learning by all parties. You may choose to channel emotion through art, or have a written 'conversation' with the other party, using your left hand for their 'voice' and your right hand for your own 'voice'. You may visualize the other party sitting in front of you while you tell them everything you need to say. You may take a HypnoBirthing® class, which includes a release of past negativity, or see a certified hypnotherapist.

You and your baby are worth whatever it takes to rise above the pain and move ahead. You must have the conviction to create what you want and eliminate what you don't. It's not your concern how this will or won't affect anyone else but you. Realize that circumstances are different now and you are in control.

CHAPTER 9

Agony or Ecstasy

Perception is reality. We give meaning to events based on our perceptions.

I was first introduced to this concept through my husband, a quality manager in the automotive industry. If the customer perceives a problem...even if no problem can be found in design or function...there is a problem. The customer's perception is the quality department's reality. Period.

The filters though which we view birthing and parenting alter our personal perceptions. This is a simple fact. Perception is reality. A dozen people can witness one event and every one of them will recount a different version of events

Two mothers can have experiences seemingly exactly the same from the outside, but have completely different internal interpretations of the value attributed to their experience.

In one video I use in my childbirth classes, one woman in labor using self-hypnosis looks like she's sleeping. Another woman in labor is howling down the hall. The birth process...the muscles involved, the action of the muscles, the birthing hormones, etc...is the same for all normal births. These two mothers are experiencing the same physical stimuli, the same sensations and functions, yet they have assigned very different meanings to their experience, thus creating different realities.

Every event in our lives is neutral, in-and-of-itself. Our interpretations are a choice. Some people tend by nature to always see the positive, some the negative. Some circumstances seem quite negative by their very nature, though we see examples all around us of people who have taken tragedy and turned it into opportunity.

It is vitally important to acknowledge that perception is reality when speaking about birth because birth is such a powerful, personal, defining moment in a woman's life. Each woman, as a unique individual, has unique perceptions, and will assign unique meaning to what takes place during her birth. Failure to understand this fully has made dialog about better birth more laborious than it needs to be. If the reader has visited birth related message boards on the internet, the truth of this has already been made apparent.

The plethora of bad birth programming on cable also illustrates this point. I find it very difficult to watch these programs because they make me so sad and angry. In one show I watched, three of three births ended up surgeries. All complications were predictable, all preventable, all caused, not encountered.

One mother was induced, labeled 'overdue' via ultrasound. The induction failed, the baby went into distress from the induction agents. Considering ultrasound is known to be an inaccurate way to assess due dates, and it is also know that inductions agents like cytotec and pitocin carry substantial risk to healthy mothers, this is not surprising.

One mother was doing great until her doctor decided she wasn't progressing 'fast enough' as per 'Freidman's curve,' meaning 1 cm per hour. The mother's doctor broke her water…again, known to be useless in substantially speeding up labor but to carry many risks. (Childbirth.org, 1998) The baby's cord washed down out of the birth canal with the tide of water rushing out, the technical term being 'cord prolapse.' Emergency cesarean.

The last mother was also doing quite well, until the nurse suggested that if the mother didn't get "her" epidural now, she couldn't have it later. The nurse assured the mother that labor would get much worse, that she shouldn't be a martyr, and that she might as well get the epidural now.

The mother, under such duress, decided to go ahead and get it. The baby went into distress, again, foreseeable. The mother was assured that the epidural had nothing to do with the series of events as she was whisked off to surgery.

In every case, cause and effect was predictable and obvious. In every case, the parents were assured the interventions had nothing to do with the complication. In every case the parents were thrilled that medical technology had 'saved' their baby. And I was furious at the injustice they'd unnecessarily endured!

This vision of birth is so foreign to what I know birth to be that I cannot fathom why anyone would willingly put themselves though this unless they were sick or injured.

Our perceptions, thus our realities, were dramatically different.

Another example is somewhat singular to HypnoBirthing.®

Many women would say that if they could envision the perfect labor it would be as short as possible. With HypnoBirthing® very short labor is becoming common. Often labors are between 2 and 4 hours and painless. Sometimes though, mothers labor for hours painlessly, not even realizing they are in labor. Or, they may realize they are in labor, but so comfortable, they go about their usual business. Then, when the fetal ejection response, a term coined by Dr. Michael Odent to describe the rapid descent a baby will make in a completely relaxed mother who is following her instinctual prompts, is triggered, the baby seems to move down quite suddenly. For some women this is uncomfortable (others actually find it enjoyable), maybe even painful, but of very short duration. The intensity may only last for a couple of contractions, or surges as they are called in HypnoBirthing, but it takes the mothers quite by surprise. Once the discomfort is felt, there may be fear that it will be so for hours more. Not realizing that birth is imminent, the mother tenses up, engaging the fear/tension/pain cycle.

It will not hinder her labor, the baby is nearly out at this point, but it will alter the experience of the event for the mother.

She may feel disappointed, even angry. If she had plans to labor in a birthing tub, surrounded by loved ones, aroma therapy, soft music and candles, her expectations have been dashed, especially if labor was so fast all she had time to do was kneel to catch a baby that was nearly falling out of her.

She may feel as if she's been 'hit by a truck' with no time to emotionally assimilate what was happening, finding herself suddenly with a newborn in her arms.

Someone who enjoyed such an experience, or someone who would like to, might respond with "Your birth was only an hour and you're upset? I'd love that!" Never-the-less, for the mother who was overwhelmed, the perception is a negative one.

Some women have been able to reframe their experience into something more positive eventually, but the fact remains their initial reactions were partly due to expectations lost, which changes the lens through which the event is viewed.

Pain is perhaps the most subjective reality of all, especially in labor. So, must pain be inherent in labor and birth?

Journal Exploration:

On the left, make a list of what you don't want. For every item on the list, create a positive affirmation on the right. For example:

I don't want a cesarean! My body is designed, and I am capable, of birthing gently and comfortably.

Then, for each item, list something that you are doing (can do or will do) to manifest what is on the right instead of what is on the left. For instance, "I will interview caregivers until I find one who supports my efforts in word and deed."

Our brains have difficulty with "negatives," so use positive language in your right hand column. What do you see in your minds eye if I say "The child did not fall down the stairs." Or, "The dog did not chase the cat." First you probably saw the child fall down the stairs or the dog chasing the cat before you could negate it. Again, for the above example, "I won't let anyone cut me!" is not appropriate, first because of it's negative language, but also because it's absolute.

Always keep in mind, the message is not to avoid technology at all costs, but only inappropriate technology that carries more risk than benefit.

Don't want: Affirmation:

What's Pain Got To Do With It?

There is no doubt that painful birth has been the experience of millions of women. So prevalent in our society is this concept, that it is taken as a given that birth must be an excruciating ordeal.

Let them cling to the notion that suffering and birthing are two sides of the same coin. I want to explore the possibility of painless birth. Without drugs.

Wait! I'm not crazy! Years ago when I first read about painless birth my reaction was also "Yeah, right!" but I've changed my beliefs regarding birth and pain. I hope I can help alleviate the fear for the reader as well.

Even in my midwifery training I learned that pain in labor is essential for both physiological and psychological reasons. I still believe that in certain instances pain is beneficial. It can be a great communicator, both guiding and warning.

I accepted without question that birth was painful. Still, I felt that it was manageable when weighed against the harm drugs posed. When I gave birth to my own daughter in 1991 labor was definitely not painless. It was bearable. I've certainly felt worse, before and since. Birth was a breeze compared to pathological pain such as a kidney infection, a ruptured ovarian cyst or a broken arm.

My own birthing experience, combined with the first hundred or so births I witnessed, reinforced my belief. I did see a couple of women give birth painlessly, one even orgasmically. However, I felt that they were lucky or somehow different from the rest of us. Maybe they had a high tolerance for pain, I reasoned.

I viewed natural birth as an accomplishment to be proud of. I marveled that there were women who trained incessantly to be thin or to climb mountains, surely enduring more pain for longer periods than what labor would require, only to demand to be numbed on the first labor twinge. I felt it quite ironic that empowerment seminars with fire walking and river rafting were all the rage, yet women's built opportunity for enlightenment was numbed with drugs. What I see now is that my belief colored what I saw, so that what I saw supported my belief.

There are known variables that contribute to pain in labor including positioning (of both mother and baby) tension, environmental factors, obstetrical management and a multitude of other things under the control of the mother. Could it be that a mother's choices, in pregnancy and during the labor and birth, had any impact on her experience? Absolutely.

Once I attained certification as a Mongan Method HypnoBirthing® practitioner and heard firsthand stories of quick and easy births over and over again, I knew for certain what I had hoped was possible. Birth isn't the problem. The obstetrically managed births, known for decades for higher morbidity and mortality rates as well as epidemically high, unnecessary surgical births, are.

It was finally the second birth of my best friend that left no doubt in my mind that my past ideas about pain in birth had been wrong.

I hoped that HypnoBirthing® would work for her. Her first birth was textbook, 12 hours of labor with 2 hours of pushing. It was hard work, and it was painful. It was emotionally difficult for me because I love her and hated to see her in pain.

When I attended her HypnoBirthing® two years later she was radiant. She was calm, relaxed and retained her keen sense of humor throughout. From the time her water broke and labor kicked in, to the time her 10 lb. 3 oz. son was in her arms, was an hour and a half with a 13-minute second stage.

As beautiful as that was, the amazing part was that she had broken her tailbone 4 days prior to birth.

She never once felt pain from her injury. She beamed, "It's over already? It was so easy!"

When I believed it, I saw it. Once I saw it, I felt compelled to understand it better.

Is Pain Inescapable in Labor?

In early attempts to let women in on the secret of comfortable birth, I asked parents in my classes if labor has to hurt. The responses have been consistent, likely thoughts the reader may have, so I will address them.

Labor Must Be Painful. It's Eve's Curse.

This belief is often attributed to the Bible, Genesis 3:16. The word translated as "pain" or "sorrow" is the Hebrew "etzev." This same word is used 16 times throughout the Bible. Nowhere else is it translated as 'pain'. In fact, in the very next verse, Genesis 3:17, it is accurately translated as it is in all other instances, as 'toil'.

Even if pain and suffering in labor were punishment for Eve's sin, isn't the purpose of baptism to cleanse away sin? Wasn't the purpose of Jesus dying on the cross to atone for the sins of the world? Many women giving birth quickly and comfortably are non-Christian. Why would they be able to birth comfortably, but the faithful suffer? How does this reasoning make a 90% epidural rate ok, but not a relaxation method for more comfortable birth?

Contractions Hurt...Everyone Knows That!

Who is 'everyone'? Obviously not all HypnoBirthing® women! Obviously not blissful home birth mothers.

The uterus contracts painlessly in it's normal functioning at times other than during birth. During menstruation, the uterus contracts,

208

the cervix opening to allow the contents of the uterus to pass. Most women will not experience pain during this process. The uterus contracts painlessly during the Braxton-Hicks contractions of pregnancy. The uterus contracts painlessly during orgasm.

Every muscle in the body functions by contraction and release. No other healthy muscle, going about its normal function, hurts. A malnourished or dehydrated muscle hurts. An injured muscle hurts. Normal function such as walking, flexing a bicep or the beating of a healthy heart does not hurt.

Something Huge is Coming Through Such a Small Opening!

The uterus is the size of a pear before pregnancy. At term, it has stretched to accommodate a small human being. Being pregnant isn't painful. There are normal discomforts as the body adjusts, but most women would not judge it painful.

The cervix has stretch receptors in it that signal the brain to release endorphins. These are the body's own strong painkillers. The cervix thins as it opens over the baby's head, as a turtleneck sweater pulled over a head. This means there is 'extra material' to work with, so to speak as it goes from very thick and soft, to paper thin, disappearing as it is taken up as part of the uterus, which it is.

Viewing images of crowning in class invariably causes wincing. Again, we look to the amazing design of women to understand why this part doesn't have to hurt.

By childbearing age, the genital area is comprised of many folds of skin. During birth, like with the 'extra' thickness of the cervix, these folds are 'taken up'. They smooth out around the baby's head until they are gone completely...like an accordion. This built in 'give' is why episiotomies are so rarely necessary.

Painless Birth — An Old-New Concept

Earlier, we explored choices in childbirth classes. A little history may shed light on how long the concept of painless birth has been around. Between the early 1900s and the 1970, three doctors tried to help American women give birth naturally and comfortably.

In 1913 Dr. Grantly Dick-Read asked a woman he'd just attended in birth why she has refused chloroform for the relief of pain. Her reply was "It didn't hurt. It wasn't mean to, was it, Doctor?" Other similar experiences caused Dick-Read to question what he'd learned about birthing. He concluded that what made these painless labors different was the absence of fear. The idea of the fear/tension/pain cycle was born. By the 1950's Dick-Read had published several books on the subject.

In the 1940's Dr. Robert Bradley became a natural childbirth proponent, coming to many of the same conclusions that Dr. Grantly Dick-Read had. From Dr. Bradley's work came his book Husband-Coached Childbirth and Bradley® Childbirth classes.

Dr. Bradley was very interested in hypnosis and originally promoted his 'method' as using hypnosis. However, during the 1950s and 1960s hypnosis was controversial. Eventually, the emphasis on hypnosis was dropped and put on "deep relaxation" instead.

During the 1950's, Dr. Ferdinand Lamaze witnessed painless birth in Russia. He documented what he felt were the essential components for a comfortable birth. In the early years, Lamaze® was unabashedly about self-hypnosis, but possibly meeting the same resistance as Bradley, his 'method' was termed "psychoprophylaxis"…or 'mind prevention'. The original intent was painless birth.

Many nurses, and doctors, object to teaching painless childbirth on the premise that if we say it's possible, women who perceive birth as painful will feel like 'failures.' In fact, right or wrong, anything contradicting current obstetrical management…much of which is the origin of pain…will be excluded from discussion.

This is like saying that if women have painful periods, they should feel like failures for not menstruating painlessly because most women do. Pain is a subjective experience. Perceptions differ. There are too many variables in birth, and in the choices that women make, to ensure that every woman have the same exact experience.

Apply this logic to any other situation and it becomes ridiculously obvious it's flawed. Say, a friend and I have two garden lots. My lot is sandy, hers rich and fertile. I have slugs and bugs, she has no pests. We have the same tools and the same seeds, but my climate is cooler for more of the year. If we plant gardens, can we expect the same results? What if I procrastinate and plant a month later than I should? What if I am guided to fertilize and choose not to? What if I let deer come in and trample what is growing?

A Rose By Any Other Name…

One mother of the 50's who had benefited from Dr. Grantley Dick-Read's work decided it was time for women to take back their births. Her name is Marie Mongan and she is the originator of a program utilizing the necessary components of a gentle birth…HypnoBirthing®.

As the name implies, HypnoBirthing® is unabashedly about self-hypnosis. Mongan has chosen to educate people about what self-hypnosis actually is instead of cloaking the method in alternative language.

Misconception still surrounds the word 'hypnosis.' It isn't something someone does to you. All hypnosis is self-hypnosis. Anyone can and does access this state several times a day. Falling asleep or waking up, driving, reading or even watching TV, our brainwave pattern is the same as in 'hypnosis'. Advertisers know this and use it to their advantage. Commercials slip information into our subconscious constantly. If we are in a state of hypnosis when a commercial comes on for a flame-broiled burger, why don't we all rush to get one?

Because no one will do something against their own values while 'in hypnosis.' Those whose only exposure to hypnosis has been stage hypnosis have probably seen participants do outrageous things, however, stage hypnotists purposely choose people who might act outrageously anyway if asked after a couple of stiff drinks.

Back to the burger…
If I am a vegetarian and a commercial comes on for a burger, I'm not going to instantly desire seared cow. I might go to my freezer for a veggie patty. However, if I'm already thinking a burger sounds good, I'll probably get up and go…or at least the thought will stick with me until the next time I drive by the burger place.

The Common Thread

As briefly mentioned earlier, in the 1970's Dr. Herbert Benson studied a state he termed the 'relaxation response'. He acknowledged that this relaxed state carried many labels, one being hypnosis. If the word hypnosis is objectionable, the physiological state and brainwave pattern characteristic of hypnosis, and the relaxation response, has also been called biofeedback, prayer and meditation. No matter what name it goes by, what's important is how the mind affects the body.

Benson's main concern was relieving stress. He recognized that modern day humans spend far too much time engaged in a "fight or flight response" which you may have heard of. His contention was that our modern life kept us in this state continually, harming our health.

In birth 'methods' that actually result in comfortable, shorter, natural birth, the interruption of the fear/tension/pain cycle was integral to the method. What I found interesting when I read Dr. Benson's work was that the essential components in what he termed the 'relaxation response,' the opposite of the 'fight or flight response,' were what made up the working 'methods' for painless birth.

The Four Elements

If we look at what is required to elicit the relaxation response, we can see why some methods may have worked when they were developed, but no longer do.

1.   A comfortable (and safe) environment.

Dr. Lamaze's concepts were difficult to implement in American hospitals where the limbic system, the primitive part of the brain that conducts birthing, interpreted strangers and unfamiliar odors as signals to 'fight or flee.' This also explains why home birth mothers usually consider their births more manageable.

Also, husband's were not allowed in the delivery room, as a rule, until Husband-Coached Childbirth. The painless births that Lamaze saw in Russia included labor support. Just this one component has since been proven to improve outcomes yet it wasn't until recent years that American women had even heard of the term 'doula' which is the term for a professional labor assistant and support person.

2.   A mental device—a sound, word, prayer, fixed gaze or focus on breathing.

The counted breath and focal point of Lamaze® is one example of this. HypnoBirthing® uses deep abdominal breathing which holds a relaxation trigger in and of itself.

3.   A passive attitude—not worrying about performing well and the ability to put aside distracting thoughts.

Again, harder to achieve in a setting where everything down to whether or not you pee enough is obtrusively assessed.

4.   A comfortable position.

When Lamaze's methods were brought over from Europe, this was not even an option in American hospitals…all women were expected to be on their backs, the most uncomfortable position imaginable for birthing.

Before the routine use of non-medically indicated technology, many of these techniques might have helped many women despite less than ideal conditions. A mother may not have been comfortable in the hospital, but she might be attended by the physician she'd had since childhood. She might not have been allowed a comfortable position, but if she were able to focus intently, she might be able to block uncomfortable sensations. As birth began to revolve around the convenience of staff and the use of technology, mothers would have had a harder time adapting. As these mothers experienced painful labors, the mothers and those attending her made the sweeping assumption that certain birthing techniques 'don't work,' never considering it was the adaptations at the level of the individual instructor, at odds with the organizational vision, that rendered it ineffective, not the method itself.

The importance of deep, slow breathing for relaxation is now widely recognized. The success couples experience is due to their dedication to being informed consumers and reducing interventions to only those that are medically indicated. Bradley,® ALACE and BirthWorks™, indeed most independent classes, help many women in the same way but may or may not teach techniques that trigger the relaxation response. HypnoBirthing® does teach such techniques along with wise consumerism.

214

New Choices

If our only choice in labor really was torture or being numb to the most important event in a woman's life, it would be quite understandable that women would disconnect. The spin that has been put on this normal process is that no drugs=pain, drugs=no pain with some serious misrepresentations. It's human nature to not look very deeply into those misrepresentations if we believe that it will take away our salvation.

Now that we know that we don't have to make a choice between suffering in labor or our babies well-being we truly have options. HypnoBirthing® has revived the concept of comfortable birth, now supported by the science of evidence based care. Those willing to conquer the fear our culture has falsely instilled in us will change the face of what it means to birth safely…gently and with dignity. We'll see it when we believe it. Perception is everything.

Everyday, in every circumstance, including the birthing of your child, you have the power to choose your perceptions. There is neither 'good' nor 'bad' sensation until you assign meaning to it. Your response to labor is not a function of physiology, but how you choose to perceive labor.

I am not suggesting that all labor is painless—only that normal labor can be. Obviously, if illness or injury should become part of the experience, pain may be an important communicator. Also, if your birthing choices include things that cause pain in labor, realistically you may or may not be able to reframe the sensation until the pain-causing elements are eliminated, either by actually removing them or by using self-hypnosis to mitigate their effect.

Do we know what causes pain in labor? Without a doubt. Anything that creates tension, fear, or disruption of the primitive birthing brain. Strangers, unfamiliar scents, bright lights, constant interruption of the mother's efforts, unnatural positions and alteration of the birthing hormones with artificial chemicals. In short, most of what is considered usual at the typical American birth today. No wonder women have a hard time accepting the idea that labor doesn't have to be painful!

If you have had a past negative or painful birth, the good news is you can choose to learn from that event, making different choices this time. Only you can decide how to use your experience. Will it continue to hurt you everyday, affecting each subsequent birth, or will you refuse to carry it beyond this day?

Emotional pain is a filter in itself. Though it may seem that it is never ending and deep, there is another side eventually. There are inspirational stories to draw from…mothers who have lost children to drunk drivers who then went on to save other's children for example. Through unspeakable pain, these individuals have made the choice to use their experiences in a positive way.

Even if you are healing from an unexpected birth outcome and it doesn't seem possible right now, there will come a time when that choice is yours. If you are pregnant again after an unfortunate outcome, as far too many wounded mothers are, it might behoove you to be courageous and seek help now before the past affects the outcome of the present.

Ultimately, how you perceive pregnancy and birth is your choice. The birth shows where strangers attend mothers in strange environments meant for sick people are alien to me. I choose to see pregnancy and birth as natural, physiological events until there is reason to believe otherwise. It's painful for me to see other people's distorted perception of birth portrayed as reality when I have seen and experienced something so radically different, especially when it's contrary to every bit of evidence as to what makes birth safe.

I understand 'perception is reality' so I recognize that the birthing choices made within such a reality make sense to the parents making them.

Our personalities, experiences, beliefs and attitudes powerfully influence the interpretations we assign to birth; those interpretations, in turn, determine what we will experience and how others will respond to us. This is neither good nor bad—it simply is. All of us view the world through our personal filters. Filters may be healthy or distorted; constructive or destructive. To make our own best decisions, we need to recognize what our filters may be so they don't distort perceptions critical to our safe birthing decisions.

There is no question that our filters include perceptions passed down to us from mothers before us who processed their own experiences through their own filters, as well as from medical personnel who view birth through the filter of pathology. A woman raised to be afraid of birth as a medical event...virtually all US women...will come to birth afraid. Fear creates pain.

If this view were reality, it would stand to reason that everyone would experience it, which we have established is not so. If there are mothers who choose a joyful experience, maybe you can consciously create a joyful reality, too!

We are products of both conscious and unconscious input. What matters is not whether that input was positive or negative, but how we choose to let it affect our pregnancy and birth now.

Maybe it's not other's perceptions that brought us to see birth as scary or dangerous. Maybe you have actually had an unfair and difficult birth. Allowing your current reality to be affected by past events allows the past to dictate both your present and your future.

In order to ensure that this baby and this birth, are not disrupted by the other, past experience, learn about what went wrong. Is it preventable? If not, is it a repeating sort of problem? Is it reasonable to be concerned this time, or is an unreasonable fear clouding your perceptions. Know your filters so you can compensate for them. Accepting accountability for what you can control in your birth makes what you can't more acceptable.

Some people adapt to stress gracefully, others come unglued when faced with the same pressures. How do they differ? One sees an opportunity, the other an obstacle. Their perceptions, their filters, determine the quality of their experience. One parent, faced with prenatal test and interventions may decide that even if the chance of something going wrong is small, they couldn't live with themselves if their child developed a problem that might have been prevented. This is actually often suggested to them by the physician who wants to do the testing. "Well, if it were my child and I could have prevented such-and-such, I couldn't live with myself." No matter if the condition of concern is likely to be minor and the treatment actually more dangerous.

Another parent might weigh the risk and benefits just as carefully and see things completely opposite. If the condition of concern is equal or lesser than possible complications resulting from the testing or treatment, this parent may say to themselves, "Of course I would feel horrible if something bad happened, preventable or not, as any parent would, but I'd feel worse it I were the one to cause it by taking the riskier action."

In the five years it took for my husband and myself to get pregnant, we did a lot of research on healthy pregnancy and safe birth. We decided that if we only got to do this once, we didn't have room for error in our choices.

After our home birth, one family member said to another, "It's a damn good thing everything turned out okay! If anything had gone wrong, I'd never forgive them!" If anything had gone wrong, which I knew to be unlikely, considering statistically I was certain we'd made the safe choice, I'm sure we would have felt sufficiently bereaved.

However, knowing what I knew about those statistics, had we opted for a hospital birth and something had gone wrong, which was much more likely, I would have felt worse because I would have felt that we knowingly put our child in danger. Ironically, we would have gotten sympathy for an unexpected outcome for the socially acceptable choice, though we didn't get support for the wonderful outcome of our socially unacceptable choice, no matter how well educated we were on the matter.

This family member loved us very much, but often, when someone else's filter is drastically different from our own, the behaviors resulting from their filters are labeled strange. Our filters were simply different.

A common misperception is that if one person's perception is right for them, the other person's must be wrong. Nothing could be further from the truth. Clearly, the perception of reality is not the same, but the reasoning behind decisions could, in fact, be very much alike. They start out with divergent filters, so their eventual reality outcome will be as well. What matters is whether or not their filters result in the safest, most satisfying birth for them. That can only be determined by each mother, each parent, alone.

The behavior of most parents, physicians and nurses would make perfect sense if the initial assumption of birth as a painful, dangerous, medical event were sound. Current obstetric management can be viewed as a test of the validity of that assumption. If pregnancy were dangerous, routine medical testing would improve outcomes. It hasn't. If birth were a medical disaster in waiting, routine medical intervention would not disrupt the process. It does. If technology were integral to the process of birth, routine technology would improve outcomes. It hasn't. If birth were inherently painful, all women would suffer without medicine. They don't. The initial assumption is proven faulty.

Continuing to behave under faulty birthing assumptions perpetuates the perception of a reality with no basis in fact. This is illogical for parents who desire comfort and safety for their birth.

Have you made assumptions regarding birth without testing their validity and then acted on those assumptions as if they were irrefutable truth? Is the consequence of this behavior that your birthing reality is based not on fact, but on a fear-based, untested perception?

If you accept the assumption that normal birth is always painful, you might disregard evidence to the contrary. This assumption will affect your opinion of women who choose to give birth at home without drugs. Your assumption may cause you to make decisions that aren't in your best interest, or that of your baby. Another woman, making the same assumption, may demand her epidural at the door. Suppose that, she too, has failed to test the initial assumption. Both of you have made faulty initial assumptions which neither has tested for truth or reliability. You may be operating logically from your perspective, but starting with wrong information, even with right thinking, can still result in huge mistakes. Your fear-based thinking is more likely to result in major complications, which will reinforce your fear...a self-perpetuating cycle. Sadly, this is where we, as women, are today. This is the cycle I want to help you break so that you, too, may experience ecstatic birth.

Unfortunately, our thinking about ourselves is most distorted by our unconscious filters. Pregnancy, birth and mothering are areas where we tend to be less objective or realistic than any other area of our lives. We completely negate the ways in which we contribute not only to our own experience of the world, but the world itself though our children. We have more resources and knowledge than our parents and grandparents had, which one would think would mean we would strive to do better by our children. Instead, I hear all the time, "It was good enough for me!" This is a defensive statement and proof of 'settling.' 'Good enough' parenting. Don't our children deserve for us to reach? Much of the reasoning behind why our ancestors did things was not based on fact. Granted, sometimes there is wisdom to be found in 'old wives tales,' but it's time to use what stands up to scrutiny and discard the rest.

It is most difficult to see our own complicity in birthing events when fixed beliefs are involved. Most of the beliefs we have about birth are fixed. Consciously or subconsciously the decision has been made to stop seeking, receiving or processing new information, making these beliefs very dangerous. If you are accepting the belief as fact, you will no longer question or modify. From this head-space, you will not only miss new data, you will fail to see anything that might negate the fixed belief. When the beliefs are ones you have about your own responsibilities in pregnancy, birthing limitations, or choices in parenting, either real or imagined, they become limiting beliefs. Limiting beliefs run rampant in the childbearing year.

One area where this has given me fits for years is pushing. For a dozen years I would instruct the parents in class to use physiological pushing. This is not what most women learn in a co-opted hospital class. They learn what is called 'purple pushing' by those of us trying to abolish this practice. It is unnecessary and harmful.

Physiological pushing basically means you do what your body tells you. It is also called 'breathing the baby down,' or 'nudging the baby out.' This doesn't mean that you never push, but that you only do if it feels good and is productive.

The natural progression of labor usually has a resting phase after full dilation is complete, yet women are instructed to begin pushing, and pushing hard, as soon as someone declares it is time through a vaginal exam. This is akin to being told to defecate or regurgitate on demand. Both of those functions require an internal reflexive prompt, as does 'pushing.' If the reflex is not there, it is a non-productive action and wasted energy to try to force it. Women being instructed to push with no urge need to be told to 'push like you're having a bowel movement' because it's the only frame of reference they have. Women who push as their bodies tell them would find that instruction ridiculous! When you feel the need to bear down, it's unmistakable, irresistible, and nothing like a bowel movement! An entirely different set of muscles is involved. When women do bear down, they don't usually hold their breath for longer than about 6 or 7 seconds, nor do they normally push three times during a one-minute surge. Holding the breath for 10 seconds, several times consecutively, restricts the baby's oxygen. Women in coma have given birth vaginally with never even pushing once! The uterus does all of the work.

However, my clients were telling me that the doctors and nurses wouldn't 'let' them conduct second stage this way. When I began teaching HypnoBirthing® I would get reports that the labor went fine…up to that point.

There is plenty of research supporting what I teach. So, I began giving a letter to my students describing what I was teaching and why, and I attached my sources so that they could share this information with their care providers. Having gotten this far in the book, you may have already guessed how much the facts changed the belief.

One nurse angrily asked me, "You don't really tell them they don't have to push do you? They have to! The babies won't descend if they don't!" Despite the fact that I gave her all of the information that I shared here, her mind was made up.

Another nurse who taught childbirth education classes (in hospital) agreed, insisting that because forced pushing speeds descent, the doctors insist on it and she didn't feel it was fair to teach something that doctors wouldn't let the mothers do. I feel differently…if I don't teach it, parents can't choose it. If I teach it, providing all of the benefits and evidence along with the detriments to their other choice, and they choose to birth with a caregiver who ignores science in an institution that doesn't honor their choice, then they have made a conscious decision to suffer a perineal laceration and to put their baby into fetal distress.

Forced pushing only speeds decent if the integrity of the pelvic floor is compromised because someone has cut into it. In that instance, yes, pushing hard will shoot that baby out. However, in a normal (read: natural) birth, think of it this way…if you have a ring on your finger and your hand is swollen, if you pull on the ring with all of your might, what happens? The tissue ahead of the ring gets in the way. Or, think of a Chinese finger trap puzzle: The harder you pull, the more it sticks.

Pushing hard against healthy, uncut pelvic floor muscles tenses the muscles and makes 2nd stage longer. Women who breathe their babies down may only feel like bearing down a few times and 2nd stage is routinely shorter with these women…often only 15 minutes or so.

If practitioners don't 'allow' passive descent because they 'know' it doesn't work (contrary to common sense, scientific evidence and the experience of women doing it) they will never see it.

These erroneous beliefs cannot be changed if they aren't acknowledged. If you don't acknowledge and identify your birth related limiting beliefs, they will actively threaten and undermine your attempts toward better birth. Often, it is when you are facing a challenge that a limiting belief will rear its ugly head, creating doubt about your ability to cope, proving fatal to your efforts. Birth is nothing if not a challenge. Neglecting limiting beliefs allows them to persist. You must confront them and eliminate them now if you want to optimize your best birthing reality.

Your objective here is to ferret out beliefs…beliefs you hold to be true and accurate, perhaps self-evident, thus treating them as fact. You no longer challenge them, if in fact you ever did. You 'know' this negative self-perception or belief about birth to be accurate so you simply accept it. Many of these are probably products of distorted cultural birth beliefs or personal filters from a past experience.

Some of these beliefs may go back as far as childhood — possibly back to your own birth. Others may be more recent or even adopted from someone else. Your limiting beliefs impact your ability to achieve your goal of better birth. Not identifying these beliefs means you are defeated before you start.

By examining the idea that certain limiting birth beliefs may be causing you to think and behave in ways that are not in your own best interest (or your baby's), you can transform you birthing possibilities. You control your attitudes and perceptions. You control what sort of birth is attainable for you. That's empowerment!

Do the required work in order to verify that your perceptions are grounded in fact. Challenge the views you hold about your mother-self and the act of giving birth instead of blindly accepting the limited perspective that holds you, and millions of other women, back and puts you at risk.

Perception is reality. Allow your perception to be grounded in fact, not myth or someone else's history. If you are using this book properly, you have already made some cognitive shifts...maybe even some spiritual shifts. Every experience, every new bit of input, can change us...better us. Let yourself be open to the growth that is motherhood.

PART FOUR
Externalization

By now you should have encountered new ideas, tested their validity and explored your feelings about how it relates to you. Now that you know you can create better birth for yourself, the next step is to seek out options available to you.

CHAPTER 10
Variables and Outcomes

We'd all like a guarantee that our pregnancies and births will go as planned. We don't get one in life, and unfortunately, we don't get one in birth. We'd like to think that bad things don't happen to good moms who make all the 'right' decisions. Realistically we know that's not always true.

So far, I've put the emphasis on how much control parents, especially mothers, have over the baby-growing and baby-birthing process. It would not be fair to imply they control all outcomes, all of the time. However, neither do doctors or hospitals. Somehow, we've gotten the impression that if we take all the prenatal tests and make sure we are in the hospital, everything will turn out right. We know this is not a reality based on fact. Even so, none of us is immune to this thinking.

Very early in a midwifery apprenticeship I attended a birth as an observer and assistant to the midwife. I was approximately 7 months pregnant. Something went dreadfully wrong. A tragic and rare occurrence, the mother suffered an amniotic fluid embolism, a rare situation (1 in 50,000) in which amniotic fluid is forced into the maternal bloodstream. It is neither predicable nor preventable. The mother was transported to the hospital via ambulance, accompanied by the midwife. The rest of us followed close behind.

When we arrived we were told both mother and baby had died. I remember thinking, as I stood there in the hall, that it just couldn't be…we were in the hospital. They were supposed to save her. That's what hospitals do. The next couple of months were difficult. I had not lost faith in birth or in my midwife. I knew there was nothing that could have been done differently.

However, in the midst of our grief for this wonderful mother, there were people with their own agenda trying to get the father to sue, trying to have criminal charges pressed against the attendants, trying to make it seem as though the fact that this was a home birth was somehow relevant to this outcome, despite the fact that same problem had occurred twice in the previous year at two different hospitals a few hundred miles apart.

In one of those other births, both the mother and baby were also lost. In the other, the baby was saved, only because the embolism happened during a cesarean and the baby had already been partially delivered when it occurred.

My first reaction, standing under those bright lights with the baby in my own belly furiously kicking from the adrenaline I was producing, was that the hospital could fix anything. That's what they are there for...emergencies. This expectation we have is not realistic, but I understand how alluring it is.

Consider a mother who loses her first born due to placental abruption; a condition wherein the placenta comes away from the uterine wall. After going to the hospital with concern over 3rd trimester bleeding and being sent home, she returns to the hospital later to undergo a cesarean of a still baby. Why surgery when the baby was already gone? Who knows? Obviously putting the mother's life at risk when there is no hope of saving the baby who was already gone makes no sense, but perhaps this idea that hospitals and surgery can fix everything was at the root of such a decision.

What makes even less sense is that for all subsequent births, this mother would have surgical deliveries before term, potentially placing them at risk for preterm complications, based on that previous event. Doctors, hospitals and technology didn't save the first baby, and in fact were responsible for the catastrophe because they ignored the mother's concerns. The unfortunate event was non-repeating, but foundational belief hospitals and doctors can assure

228

perfection, even in the face of the facts, brings us back. This is what is so perplexing when there is a (rare) home birth death and it is blamed on the birth location. Think about this. If the U.S. infant mortality rate is 6 per 1,000 (CIA, 2011) and there are approximately 4,000,000 births per year, that's 24,000 babies that die in the U.S. per year. Since most birth occur in the hospital, that's about 65 babies born in the hospital that die every day. Yet perhaps a couple of times per year we hear of a baby dying at home, and somehow people are certain it's the fault of the birth location.

We expect perfection that nature doesn't even promise. Here I'm thinking of a situation, for instance, of a mother who has a baby with several congenital abnormalities incompatible with life in which routine technology didn't predict or prevent it and could not fix it. Yet, with the idea firmly entrenched that modern medicine can give us perfect offspring, would it seem logical that this mother would ascribe the health of her subsequent children to the medical establishment? Even though, again, the condition may be non-repeating and the odds overwhelmingly in favor of normalcy after suffering such an unlikely, unlucky and heartbreaking outcome with a first baby?

Why is it that if midwives encounter similar situations to doctors, the doctors want them prosecuted...but want immunity from prosecution for themselves?

Nature has a plan. For the most part, she wants the majority of us to survive and perpetuate our species. However, sometimes bad stuff happens. Sometimes we can determine a cause, sometimes not. The more logical way to deal with those times is to prevent them when they are likely to occur, which is very rarely, but not treat every situation as if it were an emergency.

Think of how often we hear of women and babies dying in the childbearing year. Not often. We've already established that here in the US it does happen, and far more often than elsewhere.

If we adopted maternity care similar to the top 5 safest countries in which to birth, we'd hear about mother or baby deaths even less often.

"It's not an insignificant number if something is wrong with your baby" is often a comment used to manipulate parents who rely on the weighing of risk and benefit ratios in their decision making process.

Journal Exploration:

Ask yourself—and keep asking--the hard questions until the answers are clear.

What do you want and why do you want it?

What do you have to do to get it?

Are your choices based on fact or belief?

Are all of your choices in your best interest and the best interest of your child?

What must you do to get what you want?

How will it feel when you get it?

How will if feel if you don't?

How might it affect the rest of your life?

Once you know what you want and how to get it, and have set up your environment to support it, you need to let yourself believe you have a right to have it. Birth is a rite of passage that is the birthright of every woman. Be willing to allow yourself to say "I deserve this!"

No, it's not insignificant if it's your baby. No more insignificant than when a mother dies from an unnecessary surgical delivery, yet that hasn't stopped obstetricians from supporting elective cesareans. It's no less tragic when a baby dies from a hospital acquired infection that would not have happened if the baby had been born into the home in which his mother had lived, producing antibodies to pathogens she was exposed to in order to keep him safe. Yet, physicians would have us birth our babies within institutions for sick people, where antibiotic resistant organisms are a huge concern. If we are going to use the above argument in keeping babies safe, let's at least use some consistency!

We face challenges and the unexpected every day in our lives. Most of us do not live in constant fear of what might happen or what could go wrong. If we did, we wouldn't eat; we might choke. We wouldn't drive; we might be in an accident. We wouldn't take a bath; we could slip and fall. If we looked up the mortality rate for such accidental deaths, we might just find that birth is safer than things we do each-and-every day without a thought. We don't live 'just in case' lives. We take reasonable measures to avoid trouble and cope the best we can when it finds us anyway. We wear seat belts and we learn CPR. We manage.

Acceptance of this fact...taking responsibility for that which we control and accepting that which we can't...is what helps people cope when the unexpected occurs. It is inevitable that bad things will happen to some people some of the time, in pregnancy and birth as anywhere else.

With some of the challenges of birth, it is sometimes not the particular circumstance that's upsetting, but a violation of expectation. As with the mother who expects to go to the hospital to labor three hours to labor three days instead. Or, the mother who expects no pain, but ends up having a variable in her birth that makes pain unavoidable.

And the mother who eats well, gets lots of rest, carefully chooses a holistic caregiver…and ends up with a transport for a cesarean for a very real, unavoidable, unpredictable complication.

When expectation has been lost, there is grief, even if the outcome is as joyful as a live, healthy infant. As with any loss, we need to honor the feelings, not discounting disappointment or pain, then work through them and then make a decision to embrace what we have left. Only in gratitude for our blessings can we grow and heal.

The deeper losses, those of pregnancy loss or the loss of hope of a whole and healthy child, involves the same process at a much more profound level. Still, acknowledging grief and choosing to use it in a positive manner is possible. Truly, it is when we hurt the most that we are capable of anything. Many a children's hospital, cancer program or other worthwhile 'movements' have been built on a mother's grief. My own work toward better birth grew out of my desire to help other mothers have what I thought couldn't due to infertility, and then secondary infertility.

What we are focusing on here is realistic birthing expectations and emotional responses when these are not met or cannot be met. By stepping back from our culturally ingrained beliefs about what hospitals and doctors can realistically promise, we can make decisions that are based on the actual, not the potential.

Try advising yourself as if you were your own best friend, which you should be. It can be as easy to be your own best friend as your own worst enemy by simply choosing to do so. Assess your pregnancy progress and birth plans based on results, or projected results based on the probabilities laid out by statistics. These are the best predictor of future outcomes.

Ask yourself:

Is your 'best friend' (you)...

...helping you and your baby remain as healthy as your circumstance allows?

...creating opportunities for you to have a better birth?

...keeping you from making fear-based choices?

...ensuring your relationship with your partner and your caregiver nurtures you and your baby?

...requiring you to be your best mom-self for your baby?

...allowing peaceful 'down time' for you do bond with your baby and reduce stress hormones?

...providing balance and structure between work, growing a healthy baby and planning for the changes that will take place with the baby's arrival?

From this objective standpoint, are you really your best friend? Would you keep another person in your life if they treated you the way you treat you?

If another person were not treating you with the love and respect you could cut them out of your life. With great patience you must educate and motivate yourself to treat yourself better and make your own best choices.

What happens to you affects your baby, so you need to be his or her best friend and advocate too. You must treat yourself with care now and in the early years of motherhood. As my husband is fond of quoting, "If momma ain't happy, ain't nobody happy."

That is not permission for selfish behavior to the detriment of your child or partner. It's a simple principal of supply and demand. You can't nurture others if you don't first nurture yourself and allow other people to love and nurture you. In pregnancy that may mean interviewing care providers until you find one who will respect you, your intelligence and your choices. In birth, it may be insisting that your preferences be respected unless true medical indication prohibits it. In the first weeks of motherhood, it may mean putting a sign on your door telling visitors to come back when you and baby aren't resting.

Mothers deserve respect for the awesome job with which they have been entrusted. It is our duty to commit to doing it well. From the moment a woman commits to the journey of motherhood, she needs to be replenished. She is literally giving of herself. If she doesn't require the most of herself and those around her, who will?

As your own best friend, how can you create your own best birth?

First, apply everything you have learned from this book so far. It's not enough to just read it. If I told you that in 6 months I was going to take you to the middle of a lake and make you swim back to shore, but you didn't know how to swim, would you prepare? Or, would you just hope for the best?

If you only read a book about swimming, how prepared would you be? If you read a book and took lessons, how prepared would you be? If you read a book, took lessons and practiced for a few months, how prepared might you be?

I'm leading you to data, but I can't make you think. If you just read these words but don't apply the knowledge, you are no better off than when you started. Expect more from yourself and you will be amazed and pleased at how well you do.

Second, commit to resolve, rather than endure, what's not right about where you are. The longer you put up with elements of the

234

typically managed birth, the less likely you are to change it later. You must resolve to direct the greater part of your problem-solving energies toward your pregnancy and birth. It's your only priority right now. Deadlines and commitments in other areas of your life cannot compare with the life of your child. The birth of your baby, because it is a memory charged with emotion, will be a defining moment in your life, more so than any other event.

I tell the parents in my classes that the 'what if' game is a very useful tool in removing the last resistance to actually moving toward better birth.

We've all played the 'what if' game. The problem is that we don't play it right. We don't follow our 'what if' to the logical and true conclusion. Since our fears are almost always worse than reality, our 'what ifs' do more harm than good. But playing the 'what if' game a little differently allows us to work through our fears. What if the mysterious 'something' were to happen? What if something is wrong with the baby? Take any fear and make it specific. Research it. Find out if it's a reasonable thing to be concerned about or if it's an irrational fear.

Irrational fear is fear that is disproportionate to the actual risk. What is the actual incidence of the thing you fear? If it is a fairly common variation in pregnancy or birth, how often is it really an actual problem? Compare it to something that carries the same risk as in the choking example…is that something you are afraid of? Is it a variation of normal or a true complication? Are you at risk for some reason, or is this an equal opportunity complication? If you alone are at risk, is there anything you can personally do to lower the risk? Are there minimally invasive options to invasive intervention that might be suggested?

Most of the things parents toss into our 'what if' games in class are usually non-issues for normal, healthy mother-babies. For example, one that was tossed at me as a 'what if' reason that having my baby at home was irresponsible was, "What if your baby is born with the cord around the neck and the baby is strangled?" Knowing that babies who aren't breathing with their lungs yet can't be strangled by the cord made this a nonissue for me. Further, knowing that a cord around the neck is not uncommon and can be easily managed in the unlikely event it is a problem (for instance if it is short or wrapped many times) also allowed me to not be bothered by the possibility. By illuminating the shadows with the light of knowledge, we can play the 'what if game' more constructively. We can move past the debilitating fear of the unknown.

By taking the time to consider, research and actually answer the 'how' 'what if' 'why', and 'what' questions you can assure yourself that things are not nearly as overwhelming as you first imagined.
Maybe your fear is a cesarean, which is a reasonable concern. Instead of allowing your fear to manifest into reality by feeding into it, throw a little knowledge at it. What are the primary reasons behind unnecessary cesareans? Fictional cephalo-pelvic disproportion (CPD)? Failure to progress (FTP)? Questionable fetal distress, or distress caused by inappropriate technology that was ostensibly used to prevent cesarean? An emergency surgery due to pre-eclampsia from a low calorie, low salt diet that was prescribed for gestational diabetes that could have been avoided by simply not eating sugar (or not taking the test if a woman is not actually at risk)? Fill in the blank with any avoidable unnecessary cesarean set-up.

What are the real, unavoidable indications for a cesarean? A transverse baby who can't be convinced to move to a favorable position? Pre-eclampsia due to liver compromise or naturally occurring high blood pressure? Actual, pre-existing diabetes? Conjoined twins, a mother's malformed pelvis, cord prolapse not caused by artificially rupturing the membranes, or a placental abruption? Yes, bad things do rarely occur.

Can any of the bad things be prevented through excellent self-care or minimally invasive technology? Which are predictable? Treatable? For the complications that do require a necessary cesarean, how can

236

you lessen the physical challenges or emotional trauma that can accompany surgery?

Play the game to its logical conclusion. Deal with what you can, figure out how to manage what you can't.

Another responsibility you have as your own best friend, is do deal with any emotional issues in a timely manner. Believe me when I tell you that your child's childhood is no time to deal with your own childhood baggage. Children, even babies, press our buttons. Oh, not intentionally, at least for the first couple of years, but push they do.

If you have unresolved emotional conflicts, relational problems or an inability to distinguish frustration from anger, you may be apt to 'cumulatively react' to your baby's needs as expressed through his or her crying...the only mode of communication available to an infant at first. Likewise, you may react to your partners differing communication style inappropriately. Before baby, different ways of relating may not have been a problem, but after baby, there is so much more to communicate about! Miscommunication, non-communication, making assumptions or taking things personally can create huge problems in a relationship that was stable to begin with...it will most certainly end a relationship that wasn't. Now that you have created another human being that is part of your familial relationship, you have an obligation to try harder to make your union strong. Fluctuating hormones and sleep deprivation are common in the first weeks after the baby is born and tend to exacerbate any tendency to over-react if it's already present.

Invariably, at six weeks postpartum, I get calls from mothers in the midst of a meltdown. Baby has a growth spurt, mom may feel either isolated, if she's staying home, or conflicted/overwhelmed if she's going to do work other than mothering. In a moment, she looks at Dad, whose life seems not to have substantially changed and realizes...her life will never be the same. Of course this is her perspective, which is her reality, though if there is good communication she will realize Dad's life is probably going through changes as well. Life will never even be remotely similar to what it was before baby.

Mom is a completely different person. Her self-perception has shifted and her social standing has changed. She now must think for another human being, anticipating every mood and eventuality, indefinitely. Her body is providing nourishment, comfort and...well, *everything* for another person. This may lead to just not wanting to be touched even one more time by anyone else, which many women refer to as being 'touched out.' There are countless factors involved in how a parent's life changes. If unfinished emotional business and/or inadequate communication between partners is added to the mix, it's no wonder so many marriages fail soon after baby arrives.

Parents are planning (minimally, with a 4 to 6 week series of 2-hour classes, usually) for the birth, but not for life with a new family member... with individual and distinct needs.

Get closure on issues of a parental nature. Will you parent the way your parents did, or your partner's? A combination...or neither? Do you hold resentments against your parents or partner's parents? What do you know about feeding, circumcision, vaccination, healthy sleeping arrangements for baby, discipline? Do you both agree on your options? Is your relationship well grounded and healthy? Are forgiveness, apologies or confrontations required to get past certain issues?

Refuse to allow unresolved issues to burden your relationship with your baby and your baby's other parent. Whatever it takes to start out fresh, do it. Your baby deserves a clean slate.

Finally, have integrity in your word. If you've made promises to yourself, to put your baby first, take steps to keep those promises. Now is the best time to break any bad habits you, and those around you, may have developed when it comes to commitment. Actually, bad habits in general.

238

Children are mirrors, reflecting back to us both the best and the worst of ourselves.

Children are especially aware of broken agreements, spoken or unspoken. When you make the decision to bring them into the world you automatically became their safe haven. Make sure that you are. You agreed to be their protector, their provider; to teach them and to learn from them. You made a commitment to raise them in a stable environment and to put their needs before your wants. If you didn't make those commitments you had no business creating a life. Children are not a lifestyle choice. They are human beings with needs that are yours to meet. Putting anything above that responsibility tells them, loud and clear, that they are not your priority. Whether you intend it or not, they feel rejected.

That means childbirth classes come before cable and books on better birth come before a new spring wardrobe. It means you pay out of pocket for evidence-based care if you have to, even if it means downsizing a little or sacrificing some indulgence. Note that this the options are different based on different circumstances. A mother who must work two jobs just to feed herself so she can nourish her growing baby and provide a safe place to lay her head down is not going to prioritize a childbirth class over physical needs. She may, however, seek out library books on childbirth to read on her commute. We do the best with what we can from where we are at any given moment.

If you've been unreliable before, you can no longer afford the luxury of selfishness or procrastination. As a parent, you must work as hard as you would expect anyone you might hire as a substitute parent (which is what you would hope for in a 'babysitter'), and then some. Treat your new role of mother as if it matters...because it does!

Parenting is, to a large extent, a learn-as-you-go process, because you never know what lessons your little one has in store for you. Making a commitment to learn the basics will put you ahead of the game. Giving special significance to this job above all other concerns, not later, but now, shows you respect your unique status see your responsibility as important.

If you just sort of decided you wanted a comfortable, safer birth, but you never get around to finding a class, how effective have you been? If you go every week, but arrive late, disrupt class, never practice, and mock the likely effectiveness of the techniques, how effective can that class be?

Contrast that attitude with the parents who are willing to spend hundreds of dollars on a non-subsidized class and drive two hours each way to attend ten to twelve hours of instruction. The difference in the outcome that could be expected should be obvious.

Do you have a conviction that you deserve the wonderful births that others have? Are you and your baby worth the effort required to get it? Remember, the primary difference between the fairytale births and the nightmare births is that often the fairytale birthers were willing to do what the nightmare birthers weren't willing to do.

Don't sell yourself short, settling for too little, too late. Your pregnancy will keep advancing, your baby will keep growing, your due month will keep approaching—whether you are doing something to optimize your birth outcome or not. Don't promise yourself you'll do better tomorrow. Start now. Make better birth a priority and you will be far more likely to have it.

I'm not suggesting that just because you are now willing to reach for a better birth everyone will make it easy for you. You will still have hurdles to jump. It may even seem that the more you learn about your options, the harder you have to fight for the right to make your own decisions. Anything worth having is worth working for. A comfortable, safe birth and healthy, whole mother-baby are definitely worth having.

Birth and early motherhood are not to be feared, just carefully, purposely and lovingly navigated. The experiences you are about to undergo are transformative if you allow them to be…if you consciously take your turn at empowerment and even enlightenment. Standing up for yourself in pregnancy gives you strength to carry with you to your birthing. The rite-of-passage that is birth gives you the courage to love without reservation. Mother-love equips you to manage your new and ever changing life.

The tools you've learned thus far have helped you to ground yourself if you've consciously applied them. These baby steps should have minimized or eliminated many of the impediments to better birth.

Your grounded-ness stems from certain life decisions that are part of your very being. You may not consciously be aware of what these are, but they guide your actions daily. You may have made a life decision that you would protect your child with your own life. You may have decided nothing is more important than your baby. Choices you make spring from these decisions. What are your personal commitments to parenthood?

If you set unattainable goals for yourself, of course, you are putting yourself at a disadvantage. Likewise, if you don't require much of yourself, you won't get much…and neither will your baby. Be realistic in your expectations and take motherhood empowerment one step at a time. There's no better time to demand excellence of yourself. No one else can do the work you are doing.

Staying in your comfort zone now can be hazardous to your health and your baby's. You are the sole agent for change in your birth. If you don't take action toward better birth, no one else will. If you want events to progress more safely and comfortably than everyone else's births, you're the one who must make it happen.

It's not enough to change your ideas about birth, or even change what you feel…you must take action on those shifts. Remember, do what everyone else has been doing, get what everyone else has been getting.

If you want that safer, more comfortable, dignified birth, you must ask yourself everyday, "What am I doing to make my birth better?" Then, do something!

Stepping into your mother-self creates obvious changes not just in your decisions, but in your very stature, your demeanor, your speech.

You stop 'going with the flow' and become passionate about mother-love. You are your own excellence indicator. You know if you are being true to yourself or not.

Not every decision you make in your pregnancy will be great or even good. Others may not be 100% supportive. By now you should be committed to working it out and finding solutions when you make a wrong decision for yourself, making a wrong decision right.

The stakes are high…the quality of life for you and your family. Your baby's life. Your life. Your hopes and dreams. You have the skills to simply 'survive' a bad experience, but why should you settle for survival when you can have joy and wholeness in body, mind and spirit?

This isn't just your life we're talking about, but a new human on the planet. By extension the lives affected include, a father's, grandparents, siblings, teachers, friends and potentially literally thousands more if we include them any lives that one person touches in their lifetime. If each birthing woman made better birthing choices we could save our government billions of wasted health care dollars, allocating them instead to care for the sick, injured and elderly.
The danger component has been overemphasized for far too long, but now that you know that, you can move ahead with purpose and knowledge, creating a better birth…a better life.

The only promises that are for sure are the ones mothers make to themselves. The trick to managing special circumstances positively is being well grounded in the control you do have, but being flexible when the unexpected occurs. Your birthing and parenting convictions are what keeps you on track.

Journal Exploration:

Rate where you are in relation to your ideal. On a scale of one to ten, with one feeling unsure or afraid and ten being fully confident, decide if your words and actions are representative of your feelings.

On your scale, circle your ideal, then place a mark over where you feel you actually are. For example:

I know all I can know about prenatal testing 1 2 3 Ø 5 6 7 8 9 (10)
to make my own best decisions about them.

In this instance, I may not feel it's realistic to ever know enough, but in being honest with myself, I admit I haven't really made much of an effort.

Now it's your turn.

I understand the purpose behind routine prenatal testing that I am encouraged to have   1 2 3 4 5 6 7 8 9 10

I am aware of the accuracy rate of these recommended tests   1 2 3 4 5 6 7 8 9 10

I am confident my care provider uses technology appropriately   1 2 3 4 5 6 7 8 9 10

I trust that I am able to give true informed consent for recommended interventions   1 2 3 4 5 6 7 8 9 10

I have researched all viable options for safe birth locations for my situation, and have evaluated them fairly   1 2 3 4 5 6 7 8 9 10

I know the pros and cons of all of the parenting choices I will face after the birth (vaccination, circumcision, feeding, etc.)   1 2 3 4 5 6 7 8 9 10

I am aware of the importance of brain development from birth to three years, and have done everything I can to optimize my child's potential   1 2 3 4 5 6 7 8 9 10

Continue on your own. Make a list of what you feel are the ideal characteristics of a good parent. Then decide how close you are to your ideal. If you fall short, make a checklist of what you might do to bring you closer to your ideal. How many of these actions can you actually take? How might you have to re-prioritize to become a better parent? Are your ideals realistic? Have other parents been able to achieve these ideals and how did they do it? Are their situations similar to yours or can you re-structure your life to be similar to those you wish to emulate? If their circumstances are different than yours and you are unable to make significant changes, are there other ways to make your goal a reality by doing the best you can with what you have?

CHAPTER 11
Safety First!

People will treat us the way we allow them to treat us. This includes your partner, your caregiver, and eventually, your child. When preparing for a better birth, this concept is primary. The provider/mother relationship is all too often based on inequity.

This inequity is, in fact, so commonly extreme in severity that we can't even see how distorted and unhealthy it is. For example, being instructed to stripe down and gown up before even speaking with a provider during a physical, thus having to converse and ask questions while feeling quite vulnerable. Your relationship may not fall into this category, which makes you truly fortunate. Even if you feel this irrelevant to your experience, please read on. We will discuss how this same concept is at work in other relationships, including relationships with those you probably won't meet until you are in labor.

If you are going to have a better birth, you will have to negotiate, not with one person, but with many, unless, perhaps, you are birthing at home with a midwife. In that instance, negotiations will be one-on-one for the most part. At most, one or two apprentices could be involved in your birth, but only if you agree to the arrangement. At home, you should always have the final say in what you do and where you do it, unless there is a compelling reason to do otherwise, which the midwife explains to the parents.

People learn by trial-and-error, reward and punishment. We do what rewards us and avoid (or try to) what doesn't, particularly when we think we might get hurt. Except, it seems, when it comes to pregnancy and birth in the United States.

Consider the following illustrations:

Upon hearing that I was planning a home birth, one father exclaimed, "That's just nuts! We were so lucky we were in the hospital! When they broke [his wife's] water, the cord came out before the baby and our baby could have died! We were lucky the staff was there to save our baby!"

He's right; they were lucky. Cord prolapse is very serious and most often does require surgery to save the baby's life. However, his baby would not have been in danger if it weren't for the unnecessary use of a dangerous intervention, amniotomy (breaking of the bag of water) which is used so often in birth that people consider it a normal part of labor.

In the last several months I've heard of two different doctors in two different areas of the country tell women that their vaginas were damaged so badly with their first births that they wouldn't be able to have vaginal births for current babies. One doctor said this during a news program, detailing the extensive damage done to the pelvic floor with natural birth, advocating elective cesareans.

What I want to know is what they are doing to those poor women to cause such damage, because it certainly isn't part of natural birth! If a doctor is incapable of helping women deliver over an intact perineum or butchers her so badly her bottom is then useless for the most important task it was designed for, she needs to find a new provider! Yet, the women in these instances didn't even question the outcomes!

During that same time frame, a fellow childbirth practitioner had a client who was told by her doctor that she would need a cesarean because she had hemorrhoids. Certainly hemorrhoids are uncomfortable, but not an a reason to perform major abdominal surgery! It's a sad state of affairs, but there are surgeons out there looking for a reason to do surgery using the most inane excuses, and women are letting them get away with it.

246

These things continue because they can...because no one is questioning safety, efficacy or even the nonsensical nature of some of these recommendations. By allowing dangerous practices to continue unchecked, we give them permission to continue. As a society we have made a collective agreement that substandard care is okay, and that we will defend it to our very deaths.

I would like you for a moment to consider a situation that strikes me as similar.

For years, smoking was socially acceptable without question. Manufacturers touted cigarettes as beneficial. Celebrities promoted smoking. Doctors even encouraged women to smoke to help keep weight down!

Eventually, some people questioned the safety of voluntarily inhaling thousands of poisonous chemical compounds. Some people were connecting the dots between cigarettes and cancer, asthma and emphysema deaths. These people voiced their concerns. They were ignored at first. I remember the acrimonious reaction to these discoveries and announcements. "My grandma lived to be a hundred and smoked every day of her life!" or "My brother has asthma and he's never smoked!"

The evidence continued to mount. Some people quit, others rationalized. "Smoking is the only thing that calms me down" even though cigarettes are primarily stimulants, not relaxants. (ACDE, 1999) However, smokers perceive relaxation...and as you now know, perception is reality.

In any event, smoking continued as a socially acceptable practice. "If you don't like it, no one is forcing you to light up." smokers persisted. Even if smoking was dangerous, smokers were only hurting themselves. It's their body. (Full disclosure: I smoked for 10 years before I got pregnant and many of these thoughts and comments were my own.)

Except when it isn't. Next we learned about second hand smoke and how smoking affects babies before birth. Some smokers refused to believe the research. Some smokers got more considerate. Some started to see the common sense in the idea that if you pollute your body, you will get sick. Now it wasn't just your own life you could affect, but your family and even strangers.

Anti-smoking movements coalesced. Smoke-free establishments became common. The idea spread and smoke-free towns were next as people demanded that the effects of smoking not be imposed upon non-smokers. Understandably, people that had smoked for years while it was socially acceptable were irate that all of the sudden they were outcasts.

Emphasis was placed on the amount of money smokers cost our government in a variety of ways. Whistleblower lawsuits followed when it was revealed that tobacco companies knowingly and willingly contributed to the loss of billions of governmental health care dollars. Ad campaigns focused on lost wages from smoking and how smoking impacts the work place through increased sick days lost. Insurance rates were raised for smokers.

Are you wondering where I'm going with all of this? How women give birth and parent is a personal choice. It also ripples out into a larger cultural context that affects us all. The evidence against medically managed birth for healthy women is abundant. Yet, it persists because we allow it. Unless and until it is challenged it will continue…because it can.

Almost all of the societal effects of smoking can be applied to the mismanagement of healthy pregnancy/normal birth and low breastfeeding rates. I have heard it said that a parent is only as happy as their unhappiest child. I would suggest that could be extrapolated to society-at-large.

When mothers reward, accept and validate unacceptable conduct by continuing to see a care provider who abuses his or her authority,

248

they are assuring that bad behavior will repeat. There are plenty of compassionate and competent care providers out there. Reward them. Soon enough manipulative tactics and inappropriately applied technology will be as frowned upon as smoking has become.

Relationships are mutually defined. Obstetricians are the most sued profession (Greve,2009) because they have taught the birthing public that legal action is the only recourse available to rectify a bad outcome. In a power-over situation, the powerless will seek retribution in a way that gives them their power back, even if it's only momentary or superficially.

This problem is magnified in that many times, when parents decide they will no longer put up with offensive behavior from a provider, their attempts to find a replacement are futile. The other providers support poor behavior by making it difficult, if not impossible, for parents to switch. Add to this the limitations of HMOs and it seems parents are between a rock and a hard place. Is it any wonder they are angry enough to seek punishment when their instincts are proven correct and something bad happens?

We have also meekly accepted that the costs of birth require what amounts to a substantial loan. We pay a lot of money to be treated poorly!

You may never have considered that you were negotiating and creating the relationship that exists with your caregiver. After all, you may only see him for 10 minutes once per month. Now you know. Because you are aware of how your own action, or inaction, contributes to the relationship, you can choose to change it if you need to. You are the only one responsible for this relationship since you can't change a person who doesn't want to change. Why would doctors want to change the current system?

I see mothers all the time who realize this intellectually, but just keep trying to change their caregiver with every visit…instead of changing caregivers.

Albert Einstein once noted, "Insanity is doing the same thing over and over again...and expecting different results."

Women keep going back to doctors that lie to them and whose mistreatment to their bodies resulted in lifetime consequences. If you don't expect people to treat you with dignity and respect, they won't. Plain and simple.

I cringe inside when I hear birth stories full of statements like, "Then they broke my water" or "Then they put cytotec on my cervix to induce me." Where is personal accountability here? Not to mention, informed consent.

It is the law that parents understand and consent to any procedure. It is a right that carries responsibility. In order to consent, we must know if we are getting all of the information we need to decide.

If not, (and it's obvious that in most cases patients are being woefully misinformed or under-informed by the amount of harmful intervention in birth today) doctors have taken on that responsibility themselves...which is when a lawsuit may be warranted.
I have yet to see an actual epidural consent form that realistically lays out the potential risks of epidurals. However, if one did exist, it might look like this.*

*Many of these satirical forms are on the internet, but attribution is hard to come by and they are all very similar. I first found this at:
www.gentlebirth.org/archives/epdrlrsk.html with no source or author given. I would like to credit the author in future editions of this work. Please contact me if you are the creator.

EPIDURAL CONSENT FORM

1. I authorize the performance upon _____ (patients name) of the following procedure _____ (elective epidural) performed under the direction of _____(physician's name).

2. I consent to the administration of local anesthetics, narcotics, 'caine derivatives and/or other medications into the epidural space.

3. I understand that the following risks, among others, are possible complications as reported in the medical literature:

Failure to relieve pain.

Hypotension (low blood pressure).

Postdural puncture (spinal) headache which may require medical therapy.

Persistent area of numbness and/or weakness of the lower extremities.

Temporary nausea and vomiting.

Breakage of needles, catheters, etc. possibly requiring surgery.

Hematoma (blood clot) possibly requiring surgery.

Infection.

Rapid absorption of local anesthetics causing dizziness and seizures.

Temporary total spinal anesthesia (requiring life support systems).

Respiratory and/or cardiac arrest (requiring life support systems).

Back pain.

Fetal distress resulting from one of the above complications.

Permanent paralysis

Increased cesarean rate, increasing the mortality rate

Neurological damage to my newborn

Epidural fever for my newborn (requiring a spinal tap, etc.)

4. I consent to the performance of procedures in addition to or different from those above, whether or not arising from presently unforeseen conditions, which the above named doctor or his associates or assistants including residents, may consider necessary or advisable in the course of the procedure.

5. The purpose of the procedure, possible alternative methods of treatments, the risks involved and the possibility of complications have been fully explained to me. I fully understand the administration protocols of an epidural. I understand that no guarantee or assurance has been given by anyone as to the results that may be obtained.

Equal time to equal risk?

A VBAC consent form details the horrors that could befall a woman choosing this option, but there is no such consent form for cesareans. Likewise, inductions are often done without informed consent as to the probable complications associated with pharmaceutical induction agents...including the fact that they are not FDA approved for non-medially indicated inductions due to the substantial risk associated with them.

As it stands now, a parent must sign a waiver if they opt against many standard, yet unproven, interventions, but not interventions proven dangerous and/or of no use! This gives the impression that one thing is safe while another is not. Of course, this is the intent. It is subtle manipulation in action.

Analyze your own relational behavior with your caregiver. Is this a mutually respectful relationship? Is there adequate time to communicate your needs at each prenatal visit? Do you understand and accept your caregiver's limitations? Is your doctor capable of assisting a woman in birthing over an intact perineum? Does your midwife have a good working relationship with local medical personnel so that transport, should it become prudent, would be smooth? (Keep in mind all variables. I know many great midwives with wonderful outcomes who have made every attempt to establish working relationships with other professionals, but have been met with less than warm responses...to say the least.)

You can determine whether, or not, the things people do are working for you. You can change the relationship—either the agreed upon dynamics with the one you have or actually changing to a different provider. You are the only constant in this event.

Starting today, this minute, internalize the concept, that you have the power. It may not be easy, but you have to decide that you and your baby are worth the trouble.

How you respond to a caregiver's treatment of you governs your relationship. Their response to you is equally important. Resistance to your insistence of respect is a warning sign. When people get their way by controlling and manipulative tactics, they have just been rewarded for that behavior.

Notice how you feel after your next visit with your midwife or physician. Were they attentive or indifferent? Were they preoccupied with your chart or inquisitive about your life as it related to your health? Were your questions answered to your satisfaction? Was your caregiver supportive and encouraging if you sought out a variety of sources of information about your care? Pay attention to body language — did words and actions seem to be consistent? What did your mother's intuition say? If you had a similar interaction with your life partner, a sibling or co-worker, would it be positive, negative or neutrally acceptable?

This works both ways, of course. Doctors and midwives, are your clients pulling their weight in the relationship? Or, are they coasting, expecting you to be responsible for their health? Do you know if your client is still smoking, drinking or taking drugs, and if they are, do you fail to say anything or demand better? If so, you have just agreed to clean up after her mess. Failure to do so, even if it's not humanly possible, means she will place the blame on you. Don't give her a false sense of security by implying it's no big deal because you want to be politically correct. When that security is shattered, she won't blame herself…she'll blame you and she'll expect you to pay her for the pain and suffering she caused herself.

I've heard providers say that they can't demand more from their patients, or that it's financial suicide say 'no' to a client when they demand elective cesareans, non-medically indicated drugs or even antibiotics for viral infections. Even though the doctors are well aware that prescribing antibiotics for a cold will do nothing about the virus and contributes to astronomical problems with antibiotic resistant organisms.

Has this been working for them? If it was, malpractice suits wouldn't be putting them out of business. Looking at the big picture, might dropping a client who, in a lifetime, contribute a few thousand dollars to the doctors bottom line be a better choice than setting up the perfect conditions for a multi-million dollar lawsuit? Which is financial suicide?

Relationships within families and social circles also change when women start redefining what is acceptable to them regarding their birth. Many women intrinsically feel comfortable with the elements of a safe birth...good maternal nutrition, midwifery, natural childbirth, home birth and breastfeeding.

They would choose midwifery and breastfeeding because it makes sense to them right down to their bones. They are sure enough about their convictions that they could change care providers—if they had support. They go home from a visit with a midwife excited, only to have their husband 'put his foot down' and insist on all the bells and whistles of a medically managed birth.

This relationship needs redefining. Communication needs to be clear and explored in a calm environment. Ideally, it took loving cooperation to get the baby in there, ideally that's what it takes to birth it gently.

Mothers need to actively listen to what their partner is saying. Usually, a father's objections to unfamiliar birth options are just that...objection to the unfamiliar. They have grown up with all of the fear and misconceptions about birth that women have...with no intimate knowledge of women's 'mysteries' or inner knowing. They want to protect their partner and baby. Machines and external references to the unknown feel safe to them. In return, fathers must listen to what the mothers are trying to say, instead of insisting on the last word when they know little to nothing about the subject.

Agree to learn about your options together. If one of you has more knowledge about safe birth, help educate each other. Tell him you are perfectly willing to do things his way if he can demonstrate that his way is supported by evidence. In situations where mothers have lovingly shown fathers (and grandparents!) the merits of home birth, those who were resistant have subsequently become the strongest advocates!

Early in my teaching career, there was a mother who wanted a home birth. She had strong faith in the birthing design of women. She had two previous births that were somewhat traumatic. She had a strong intuition that the complications she experienced were iatrogenic and she was right.

The father feared for his wife's safety, but attributed the problems in the previous births to birth, not obstetrically managed birth. He was a loving and wonderful husband, willing to learn all he could, but just could not get 'on board' with the idea of home birth.

He was willing to compromise by getting a doula or labor support person to stay at home as long as possible, going in to the hospital for the actual birth. Throughout that birth, he was very sweet, asking often if it was time to warm up the car. He repeatedly suggested maybe it was time to get going. She labored beautifully. He wanted to help her birth her way, but it was obvious he was nervous. She went in to the hospital at 7 cm dilation, had her baby and returned home after a few hours of observation.

With the next baby, he was more willing to consider home birth, and did extensive research. His confidence grew as his wife's gorgeous belly grew. Their home birth was a family event, full of love and support. They've gone on to have another baby at home since. The initial resistance of the father and medically oriented family members has melted away.

Mothers have interviewed HypnoBirthing® practitioners thrilled with the prospect of comfortable, fast labor, only to have their siblings or parents influence them against it later. This might be due to their own ignorance about safe birth, or it may be that they see an alternative approach to what they might have done as threatening. This would be especially true if they have seeds of doubt about their own choices.

Parents must be patient, but firm, about their choices in this circumstance. If others can contribute in a positive way, let them know you are grateful for their help. If they are not supportive, ask them what they actually know about the options you have chosen. You know they have your best interests at heart, but are their ideas based on fact? If they make claims, assertions or statements, ask them to substantiate them. You'll find, after having gone through this book, that their concerns are most likely based on unfounded fears and beliefs they regard as facts. Take the time to help them though these issues the way this book has helped you. If they are unwilling to explore their beliefs, you may have to limit the input you are willing to accept from them.

Besides family, friends and even strangers may inundate you with horrible stories, criticism or unsolicited (and bad) advice. It's okay to politely stop them, thank them for their concern and inform them that you prefer not to hear such negativity. Pat your belly, smile, and tell them "especially with little ears listening." If you can educate them and get them beyond their own fear, wonderful. If they are simply acquaintances and not worth the time and effort it would take, let them deal with their own birth issues on someone else's time.

Your commitment to positive action must come from a place of strength. If you have self-doubt or fear because you haven't come to terms with the truth about birth, you won't have the ability to stand your ground. If you haven't worked through your fear by now, you may need to go back and see if you've been completely honest with yourself in previous journal explorations. Childbirth education programs for better birth have encountered situations in which women claim they 'don't work'…when the women have never even opened the book or done the work in the class! Talk about denial! How is the class supposed to work? Magic?

If you have done the work, those around you must be clear that you have not adopted your new birthing attitudes for shock value or because it's 'in.' You are now making decisions for the safe arrival of your baby. You are making decisions that ensure you and your baby are treated with dignity and respect for a healthy, happy outcome.

Don't be tempted to play the victim. I have heard "I really wanted a home birth, but…" followed by some excuse that blames a husband or insurance company, followed by a sad birth tale. Once, a woman who had expressed interest in home birth before becoming pregnant, insisted once she was pregnant, that she had chose a hospital birth because her husband had diabetes! How is this relevant? Well, the logic was that home birth would stress him out and stress altered his blood sugar levels, so it was for his safely, you see, that they needed to be in the hospital.

The funny thing is, she came up with this bizarre rationalization as if it matters to me where she gives birth! I do get exasperated when I encounter situations like these. It's inconceivable to me that women intentionally (for once someone has suggested the risk, it takes intention to avoid looking into the claim, either to prove it wrong or prove it right) and willingly put themselves and their babies in harms way under the delusion that they are doing exactly the opposite.

A mother who really wants a home birth (or any other birth) will find a way to make it happen. If you don't want one, fine! Say so. You are responsible for your own decisions whether you face that fact or not, which includes the outcomes attached to said decisions.

This responsibility extends to the hiring of a doula as well. Your relationship with a labor support person needs to rest on the same principals of trust and good communication that all of the previously discussed relationships rest.

There is one relationship that may end up as part of your experience, if you choose a hospital birth that cannot really be assessed beforehand. This would be with the nurses that will assist you throughout most of your labor.

Most of the time, you will not meet the women (or men) you will share your labor with until you are admitted into their care. Negotiation of these relationships occurs in an accelerated fashion, with unique stressors providing a great degree of difficulty.

In labor, at some point, you are in a very suggestible state akin to self-hypnosis, whether you intentionally use self-hypnosis or not. It is a natural state-of-grace we get if we go with the flow of labor. Even if we don't, we reach it eventually…through exhaustion if we have entered the fear/tension/pain vortex.

WHEN YOU WANT TO BELIEVE IN SOMETHING, YOU ALSO HAVE TO BELIEVE IN EVERYTHING THAT'S NECESSARY FOR BELIEVING IN IT.
UGO BETTI
STRUGGLE TILL DAWN

The vast majority of nurses are kind souls who care very deeply about women and babies. Because of the very nature of their work in places of the sick and injured, they view birth as pathology…or potential pathology. They may care very much, but they still operate under a certain birthing paradigm that may be very different than your own.

Open-minded nurses working from a neutral paradigm, as well as nurses hostile to all new and different concepts, are working in obstetrical wards all over the country. You have to be ready to deal with what you get.

I have met nurses who were downright abusive, brusque and rude. I have also met angels of mercy with midwives hearts, so kind and compassionate I have waited for them to come on duty before taking a labor support client into the hospital. These nurses follow protocol—just barely.

They bend the rules when they can, pleading your case and stepping in with minimally invasive labor support techniques if they see you need help or are heading in the direction of cascading intervention.

Some nurses do everything by the book with no regard to common sense. One nurse, after a birth I attended as labor support, kept insisting after the birth that the breastfeeding mother needed to switch her baby to the other breast to avoid sore nipples. The mother explained that she had been nursing children continuously for the last 6 years and sore nipples were not an issue. The nurse just did not comprehend that the mother didn't get sore nipples, or it seems, that she could have lactated continuously through three children, and got noticeably agitated that the mother was not following her instructions.

The best way to enter this relationship is with positive expectations…with contingencies for negative reactions. Dad or a birth partner can plan to run interference if it becomes necessary. That's one reason it's important for him to be as educated as you are. Otherwise, he'll have no recourse but to acquiesce to authority. Feeling unsure, he could end up an accomplice to coercing you into care you do not want or need.

In writing your birth preferences, also called a 'birth plan,' use positive language, thank them for sharing your birth and let Dad briefly explain your birth philosophy. If you are met with an arrogant attitude of 'Okay, if you think that will work…but call me when you want to beg for your epidural,' you know you need to make a strong stand for your birth.

If a nurse dismisses your preferences, ignores your requests or makes fun of your plans, politely remind her that unless there medical indications to alter them, these are your intentions. If she is still recalcitrant, ask for another nurse. Nurses are people too, with all of the same tendencies of anyone else. There is the possibility that someone with that negative attitude could act vindictively. It's rare, but it happens. You can't know if it will happen to you until it's too late. This may be a day-job to her, but it's the birth of your baby. You deserve to be treated like the Goddess you are!

How many 'yes' responses did you have in the previous exercise? If there were more than 5 you have serious inventory to take. Are your 'yes-es' confined to one particular person, or many? Do you see a pattern of acquiescing due to a fear of authority or a fear of hurting someone you love? How can you establish (or reestablish) healthy boundaries? How might requiring more of yourself and others alter your relationships?

No one likes change. The people around you are no different. When you begin to relate differently to them, they will try to pull you back to what seems 'normal' and comfortable to them. They may be angry. They may make assumptions and take things personally. They may insist these notions of painless birth are the illusions of fringe groups and that the idea that obstetrically managed birth in America could be less than ideal is just so much garbage.

Any attempts to create doubt or guilt, or to put you on the defensive, need to be seen for what they are…desperate. There may be a manipulative attempt to dissuade you from this 'craziness.' To bring you back in line with what 'everyone else does.' There may be accusations that you are being selfish, reckless or difficult.

Stand your ground, Mother Bear. With scientific evidence and common sense behind you, ask them to prove you wrong. They won't be able to, and in the process of trying will end up educating themselves. There are plenty of supportive resources for evidence-based care and the midwifery model. Find them and you will also find other souls committed to excellence…like yourself.

While you are examining other people's motives, examine your own. Remember…what comes around goes around. If you have loving support and a care provider who is open to change, do you show gratitude? Do you have unhealthy behaviors for which you are rewarded by others? Are you holding yourself accountable for your actions? Be willing to put our own behaviors and motivators under the same scrutiny of inspection you apply to others in your quest for your best possible birth.

CHAPTER 12

To Forgive (not forget)

Birthing should be our most fond memory in life. We are meeting this new little being that has the potential to help us think, feel and act as better people in the world.

Instead, far too many women feel anger and resentment regarding their births. Women's souls are wounded every single day when violated and dis-empowered during their births. Babies suffer innumerable indignities in a system that views them as commodities instead of tiny beings with feelings.

In reading this work, there undoubtedly will be women who have 'stuffed' their 'unacceptable' feelings who now see clearly that those deep emotions are justified.

Anger and resentment—no matter how warranted—won't change the situation for the birthing mothers to come. These feelings are not helpful to the poor mothers who struggle with them.

The only way to rectify the situation, healing the hurt and helping the mothers who will birth after us, is to take back your power from those who have damaged you. It's time to take back our births!

That may sound like a battle cry, however, I don't feel women are yet in a place for a warrior approach. Books like *Silent Knife* (Wainer, Estner, 1983) and *Immaculate Deception* (Arms, 1994) are the words of warriors, vital and important, that have galvanized many women...but not every woman has a warrior spirit. Not every woman is strong enough to claim her anger. Countless women have been convinced they have no right to be angry, while others are simply unaware of how much has been stolen from them.

Still more feel the pain of knowing deep in their bellies that something wasn't right about their births, but feel powerless against what Robbie Davis-Floyd (medical/cultural anthropologist) in has called *Birth as An American Rite of Passage* (2004) the priesthood of medicine. Their trepidation is well placed. Fighting back has been fruitless so far. The powerful are only using more force to keep their power.

Though the situation is said to be a 'health care crisis', the headlines may give us the first clue that what we face isn't so much about health care as it is about money, and it isn't so much about women as it is about OB-GYNs. "Fed-up obstetricians look for a way out," says USA Today (Rubin, 2002) while the subtitle to the Nightly News explains, "Doctors say malpractice insurance rates are forcing them out of business." (NBC, 2002)

Before we can begin to understand why this situation is not a crisis, but an opportunity, we first need to look at the current general understanding of the problem.

The American Congress of Obstetricians and Gynecologists (ACOG), a trade organization akin to a union for obstetricians, (Wagner, 199) has issued a national 'Red Alert' on the condition of obstetrical care in America. They are correct; it is scandalous that we have some of the highest cesarean rates and some of the poorest outcomes for both mothers and babies.

However, that isn't the concern of ACOG regarding the 'Red Alert.' They are referring to obstetrician's inability to make money because medical liability rates are so high that doctors are simply unable to practice anymore. The contention is that fundamental problems with the medical liability system are to blame…if doctors weren't sued so much, we wouldn't be in such a mess. This, they explain, jeopardizes the availability of physicians to deliver babies in the US. Their solution is not to determine why obstetrics is the most sued profession, but to lobby nationwide damage award caps.

For the average person presented with this version of the story, maybe that solution makes a lot of sense.

This is a band-aid solution to a hemorrhage. Sure, it would make malpractice rates more affordable for the doctors, but the root cause of high malpractice isn't addressed. What is the real reason for high malpractice suits? Are lawyers running amok? Is the inappropriate use of technology causing more harm than good? Have OBs implied an ability to 'deliver' what nature cannot—perfection—and are now reaping the results of such hubris? Is it due to generations, now becoming parents, raised on an attitude that abdicating responsibility is a way to free one's conscience? What about true malpractice? In cases of true malice or negligence, what recourse should a parent have?

The model for reform that AGOC proposes has origins in California, where we are assured it 'works.' Works for whom? Are we to assume for mothers and babies?

In California at Madera County Hospital, during a three-year experiment in which midwives managed the vast majority of births, the neonatal death rate was reduced to less than half of what it had been for the obstetrician managed births. The California Medical Association opposed the program and it was subsequently terminated. OBs again assumed control of births, and over the next 2 ½ years neonatal death rates tripled. (Robbins, 1996)

Poor outcomes provoke lawsuits. Is it any wonder California would initiate tort reform to place a ceiling on damages that can be awarded to parents who see no alternative but to seek compensation for their pain and suffering that was, in all probability, avoidable? Are we to believe that parents consider such reforms 'successful?'

The reform proposed is predicated on the assumption that the United States is one of the safest places to give birth due to the plethora of modern technology used. Which you should now know is not true. If it were, simply limiting the dollar amount parents of damaged or dead children could collect would be a workable solution. If the resolution of our 'health care crisis' only means making sure obstetricians are adequately paid, then certainly ACOG's recommendations are the answer. If, however, the objective is to make maternity care in the US safer, as the ACOG spin implies in the media coverage, first we must address the false assumptions the public has about the state of US obstetrical care.

Some people might be surprised to learn that there has not only been no reduction in the maternal death rate in the U.S. since 1982, the maternal mortality rate has worsened. (Singh, 2010) This, when many of the current routine interventions that people tend to think save lives have been in common usage. However, if we consider that birth technology meant for sick others is not only not useful to healthy mothers, but in some cases proven harmful, (Strong, 2000; Enkin et al,1995) this trend makes sense.

It seems to me, an educated lay-person, that even if the problem were as simple as outrageous insurance premiums due to out of control litigation, the solution would be to find out why there is a problem and fix it.

So, is ACOG's solution to reduce cesareans by adopting the proven midwifery model of care? No. In fact, ACOG resists well documented proposed improvements in US maternity care (such as a midwifery based system). Why?

The problem is far more complicated than doctors facing high malpractice rates. While targeting the real source of high malpractice is imperative to the solution, it is not the solution.

It has been argued by some that lawsuits are not the appropriate way to solve the dilemma of negligent or abusive practices. It is too little, too late. Not only that, but it punishes the competent OBs (and their clients) as well as the incompetent. All of this is true, but what is the alternative?

We need to become knowledgeable consumers for the sake of our babies. We need to move from a system that punishes everyone, to a system that rewards the greater good.

The ultimate solution needs to incorporate all of the above elements: revamping US maternity care to mirror successful midwifery systems already in existence, establishing cooperative care with ethical and competent obstetricians, and helping mothers to understand the powerful position they occupy in this new triad so that they can affect change before, instead of after, damage occurs. We also need to just accept the fact that doctors are people and people do, on occasion, make mistakes. Somehow, our culture has gotten the idiotic idea that if something bad happens to them, someone always owes them money. Doctors have bore the brunt of this thinking and it must stop.

So much of the technology that is used inappropriately is used in the name of defensive medicine. Sometimes bad things just happen. Sometimes bad things even happen because parents make bad choices.

The erroneous beliefs of our birthing system also support a group of professionals whose service is integral to the future of safe maternity care, yet changing how we see birth would necessarily, and substantially, change how we view the profession of obstetrics. A collaborative relationship is imperative for safe and effective care.

Hospitals should be available in the capacity that hospitals are available to people in all other areas of healthcare....for the sick and injured. Meaning that only medically indicated technology would be covered by insurance and government programs. Any technology or treatment not scientifically proven in efficacy or safety could still be accessed with the same ease as now, but would be paid for by the parents out of pocket.

With some adjustments to the current system, cesarean rates would go down, more women would start to tell of their empowering, joyful births as precious few mothers do now and mothers could bond with their babies more fully which would lead to higher breastfeeding rates. The amount of money our country could save in healthcare costs from these changes is staggering. Combined hospital charges for birthing women and newborns totaled more than 79 BILLION dollars in 2005 and far exceeded charges for any other condition. (Sakala & Corry, 2008)

Supporting all safe options in birth is important in a free society. Just as important is ensuring that all options are safe. Our babies depend on us to make decisions for them that will determine the quality of their lives. The least we can do for them is know what the truth is and be clear on why we are making the decisions we do. Is it from a place of informed consumerism and honesty...or fear and misinformation?

An even harder question is: how we can change a system that doesn't want to change?

I say it begins with forgiveness. I don't believe all of this is happening because of some sweeping generalization that all obstetricians are bad. I do think many of them are very afraid. They understand how powerful mothers could be if they knew that they held all the cards. By keeping women afraid, they make themselves indispensable, and, so the thinking goes, if they can limit damage awards or restrict the availability of the competition, they can remain 'safe'.

Success is based on results. Their strategy is not working. Their fear of lawsuits, and the defensive medicine that stems from that fear, is only drawing to them more of that which they fear.

It's time to stop this madness. We need to call a truce amongst all parties and devise a plan that will work for everyone.

I propose that the only way to do that is through forgiveness. Anger, blame and mistrust are only hurting those that harbor and feed them. They change who we are, how we perceive the world and how we relate to others. These ugly emotions, no matter how justified they may be, affect us physically as well. Anger and fear both trigger the fight or flight response. Stress hormones, like adrenaline, flood our bodies. These stress hormones do cross the placenta and affect the delicate balance in the baby's brain development. These hormones in birth are counter-productive to birthing hormones, creating pain.

Despite the known effects of stress, mothers are 'tested' incessantly with very little positive return on the effort, quite possibly causative in the rise in postpartum depression due to the stress it creates.

In reality, some postulate, what we seem to be seeing is actually post-traumatic stress disorder (PTSD), not postpartum depression (PPD). Would that be a reasonable conclusion to draw? Let's look.

PPD symptoms:
Persistent sadness or depressed mood, loss of interest in ordinary activities, including sex, decreased energy, fatigue, lethargy, sleep disturbances (oversleeping or insomnia), weight gain or loss, lack of concentration, feelings of guilt, hopelessness, worthlessness, suicidal thoughts, irritability and agitation, excessive crying, aches and pains that don't respond to treatment, drug abuse

Some PTSD symptoms:
Inability to control emotions, difficulty managing anger, self-destructive or suicidal thoughts/behaviors, chronic pain, sexual dysfunction, panic, chronic guilt, shame and self-blame, feeling that you are permanently damaged, feeling ineffective, feeling nobody understands you, minimizing the importance of trauma, adopting distorted beliefs about the perpetrator, yourself and what actually happened, idealizing the perpetrator, inability to trust, despair, hopelessness

Not only are the PTSD symptoms eerily similar to the PPD symptoms, but the symptoms listed under PTSD that are absent from the PPD list are actually common to women suffering from PPD. Aside from the research suggesting an overabundance of pitocin (synthetic oxytocin-a nearly universal, and usually unnecessary, obstetrical intervention) has something to do with PPD, the victimization that PTSD sufferers endure is strikingly similar to women with PPD.

I also have to wonder how much misplaced anger plays into PPD? How many have heard new mothers exclaim, as I have, that they are mad at their babies for 'what he did to me' or 'what she put me through', because they erroneously attribute their problems to the birth of that baby. What they are really angry about is the management of their birth that made it traumatic.

Between the anger, the disconnect that occurs with the disruption of birth hormones in medicated/obstetrical births and sleep deprivation, is it surprising that we are seeing more child abuse as well? Motherhood is challenging enough without added stressors and removal of nature's coping mechanisms!

Since perception is reality, the victimization so many women feel in their births can transfer into all areas of their life. This feeling of powerlessness can elicit fear. Fear is often experienced as anger. This means millions of mothers have a perception of reality altered by these emotions.

A central moment in the life of a woman…that of birthing a child, an act of co-creation with the Divine, is now contaminated, eroding the quality of your emotional and relational life.

In order to ensure that your relationships with your partner and baby (or babies) are not compromised, you must realize that just because you have a right to be angry doesn't mean you have to be. Women who have been harmed by their perceived protectors, maternity care providers, must have the courage to cleanse their hearts and minds of resentment and anger.

Learning how to counter the fight or flight response with the relaxation response early in pregnancy will help you become familiar with the physical difference in how these two responses feel and can only benefit you and the baby.

You cannot give pure, unconditional love if what is in your heart is contaminated by negative emotion. Your baby deserves unadulterated love. You deserve to feel that love for yourself. Forgiveness is the key.

This may seem difficult if your idea of forgiveness requires that the party who hurt you feel remorse over their deed. Forgiveness is not contingent on closure and/or acceptance of responsibility by another party.

First of all, as we've already established, you can only change yourself. You can't change a person who doesn't want to change. Our obstetrical system—and the people within it—don't want to change. Why should they? They have the 'market' monopolized. They have legislation in the works that allows them to cause unlimited damage with impunity. They are accountable to no one and are self-regulated. They aren't required to justify 'standard of care' with evidence, nor are they required to explain why standard of care is substandard care.

Second, the primary motivational factor in obstetrics is fear. Fear of litigation and fear of 'something going wrong' (which leads back to the first fear) due to a mindset of birth=pathology.

Finally, the rest do what they do because of this belief that birth is a dangerous medical condition. Why would they apologize to anyone if they honestly feel they are just helping? They are doing the best they can with what they have.

As we established early on, every action that comes from a faulty core assumption is then flawed to its very core. The facts prove the limiting beliefs—the core assumptions—are wrong, but don't confuse them with the facts. We've already seen you can't change a belief with facts.

No one is going to apologize for the unnecessary deaths of mothers and babies. No one is going to apologize for rectoceles or the divorce resulting from a failed sex life stemming from an unnecessary episiotomy. No one is going to apologize for the brain damaged babies suffering 'birth trauma' that had nothing to do with Nature's birth design. It's unrealistic to expect an apology for the hysterectomies performed as a result of the use of pitocin or cytotec. It's simply not going to happen.

Some care providers honestly don't understand the depth of your suffering. Some make a very conscious choice not to see it. Sadly, some don't care.

Regardless, forgiveness isn't about them. It's about us. It's about healing ourselves, choosing to let go of the anger, and accepting responsibility for our own complicity in the hurtful event. It's about refusing to allow the moments of a single event to destroy every moment that follows. It's about putting safety first.

Forgiveness means letting go of expectation that the other party be involved in the healing, but more than that, it means forgiveness of self if we are to own our contribution to the painful birth experience.

That does not mean placing blame on ourselves. It means accepting that you made the choices you made in your birth. If anyone 'did' something to you, face the fact that you allowed it. You chose the consequences when you chose the birth location, the care provider and each intervention.

It may not be fair that bad things happened, especially if you are thinking "...but I didn't know I had a choice!" Unless your last birth was more than 20 years ago, the information has been easily available. Up to 20 years ago, it was available to motivated seekers. It took a choice to not know.

272

I am aware that it's not easy to accept this idea when we've been conditioned to decry such a comment is 'blaming the victim'. There obviously are other situations in which a mother has no control, no choices, no options. Mothers of 30 or 40 years ago, before the research and the information age, may have been victims. Everyone else made the choices that led to the consequences.

Every non-medical intervention—from breaking of the water to giving medication to cutting healthy tissue for no valid reason—is legally considered assault if you don't give consent. Anything inserted into the vagina is legally rape—unless you consent.

Think about how often we don't recognize this when it comes to birth.

"I wanted a home birth, but my husband wouldn't let me."
"I wanted a midwife, but my HMO won't cover it."
"Then my doctor broke my water." (or "gave me" or "made me")

Some readers may conclude that by this assertion even more obstetricians should be sued. This would be a faulty conclusion! Lawsuits are not the answer if they push doctors to practice defensive medicine, which is already part of the problem and it would only be worse we legal action increased. However, preemptively curbing the overuse and misuse of technology through education and taking back our power could result in massive change within the system.

Still, we are left with thousands, if not millions, of women who still feel the pain of having been misled or manipulated into inappropriate technology that resulted in emotional, if not physical, pain. How do we move forward and yet honor the suffering of these women? How do they heal?

Forgiveness. There is empowerment in forgiveness.

Real forgiveness is not about the perpetrator of the harm. It is about you. Forgiveness is about how you will react to an event or behavior; how you will choose to feel. It means doing what you must to preserve your own emotional well-being. It means not giving away your power. It means releasing fear and negativity and refusing to carry what isn't yours to carry. It doesn't matter if anyone else agrees to acknowledge the problem or not. What matters is that you put it down and walk away. If you don't, you allow the other person control over your life each and every day.

If you understand that you don't need the other person's cooperation — that they don't need to apologize or even know about this act of forgiveness — you can turn something painful into an impetus for positive change. It's about you, not them. It's your choice. It's a birth-day gift to yourself and your baby.

PART FIVE

Realization

ALL COMPONENTS COME TOGETHER IN THE REALIZATION
OF YOUR OWN BEST BIRTH! YOU'VE DONE THE INNER
WORK AND YOU'VE SET UP THE SUPPORTIVE CONDITIONS
FOR YOUR BIRTH IDEAL TO MANIFEST. THE COMBINATION
OF MOTHER'S INTUITION, WOMAN'S WISDOM, NATURE'S
DESIGN AND APPROPRIATELY APPLIED TECHNOLOGY
COME TOGETHER IN THE BEST WAY POSSIBLE.
HAPPY BIRTH-DAY!

CHAPTER 13

In Control

I had an epiphany the first time I heard Dr. Phil say, "If you buy the ticket, you take the ride."

Over the years I've seen numerous parents make the effort toward better birth with a strong desire and heartfelt changes, only to have it come apart at the seams. Why? Two reasons, mainly.

One, they are making decisions they know with their heads are right, but their hearts are afraid to believe more is possible. Beliefs, unconscious fears and faulty assumptions lay in wait for a moment to spring up. Modern obstetric care seems to have a justification for everything, which gives ample opportunity for doubt to creep in.

A mother is encouraged to have an ultrasound at 8 weeks. She's hesitant, having heard there could be risks to early ultrasound including increased miscarriage, but her nurse-midwife tells her that they have to determine a due date. Not knowing that a.) a due date is irrelevant at this point b.) a due date should really be a 'due month' and c.) this will do nothing to change her care, she agrees.

She is told there is 'something possibly wrong with the yolk sac' and she will need another ultrasound at 12 weeks. If there is 'something wrong with the yolk sac' she will probably miscarry. If she doesn't, a resulting anomaly could be serious enough she might be counseled to abort. If she chooses not to, nothing can be done to rectify the situation. So, either way, her care doesn't change.

It sounds as if there is medical justification, but there is none other than the concern her care provider has regarding liability. There are certain procedures and protocols (in fact most of those regarding hospital birth) that have nothing — not one thing — to do with actual safety and everything to do with the advice of a lawyer.

Consider a woman having had a previous cesarean for a failed induction. Her doctor insists that 'for her safety' they will have to induce this time if she goes past her due date, if it looks like the baby will be big (via ultrasound, of course, which can be two pounds off in either direction!) or if she doesn't deliver during daylight hours.

Despite that fact that none of these recommendations are evidence based and in fact the induction is refuted by the very study often cited as the reason for the recommendations. (Mona Lydon-Rochelle et al, 2001) This study says not that VBAC is unsafe, but that chemically induced or augmented VBAC is unsafe. But the mother in our example is convinced that she should concede. After all, it sounds like there is a medical indication. This is a case of CYA on the part of the hospital, not mom's concern.

A birth story passed my desk of a woman who was induced because her doctor thought she 'looked ready' and by ultrasound her baby looked to be about 8 ½ pounds, which he deemed to be getting 'too big.'

After sufficiently frightening her with dire predictions of a stuck baby, she consented to an induction. The parents felt the doctor was wonderful throughout the whole pregnancy and didn't feel they were pushed into induction at all. As far as the parents were concerned, the doctor was just doing his job and looking out for their best interest. Never mind that induction is notorious for ending in unnecessary cesareans (Wilson, Effken, & Butler, 2012; Ehrenthal, Xiaozhang & Strobino, 2010) without improving outcomes or that ultrasound is notorious for being highly undependable at weight estimation.

Her baby is born after a difficult labor (again, a known consequence of induction) weighing in at only 6 pounds 10 oz., under 19 inches long, with an estimated gestational age of 35 or 36 weeks. This prematurity was not only preventable, but created by the provider. The parents will be lucky if there are no developmental delays for their child, which is the reason we purport to try to prevent premature births.

Another case of preventable prematurity touched on earlier was the woman with twins. Her doctor had warned her throughout her whole pregnancy that she should expect to deliver early. By the time she was 30 weeks along, she was told she 'might not make it to next week.'

Always, the parents are making decisions based on one source of information that is hardly unbiased. It sounds as if there's medical justification, but is there? In pregnancy more than anywhere else it's important to seek out other sources of information and second opinions, yet it is precisely here that such investigation into your own health and well being is most discouraged. Why?

Chapters leading up to this point have laid out a plan for avoiding the pit falls the above parents encountered, so you are one step ahead in this area. But what of those parents at the beginning of the chapter who tried so hard and were still sabotaged? What is the other reason the best of plans were ruined?

They were trying to fit a square peg into a round hole. This behavior comes from underlying fear, the 'just in case' mentality, but it's the act of trying to make the medical model fit the midwifery model – or maybe even thinking that it's possible – that creates problems.

It sounds something like this: 'I know birth is a healthy, natural process, but [now ignore that and listen to what I really believe] we want to have our first baby with Dr. So-and-so, just in case something happens." Thus, ensuring 'something' will happen, simply by the law of probability.

It usually plays out something like this:

Mr. & Mrs. Anybody are enlightened and intelligent expectant parents. They have read a dozen books and are in an independent childbirth class. They learn about informed consumerism, evidence-based care and the consequences of inappropriate birth technology. They make a birth plan. They outline all of the things that are important to them. They take it to their doctor, who barely glances at it and says "Yeah, sure, whatever you want...as long as there are no problems." Sounds reasonable so far, right?
Mr. & Mrs. Anybody know that midwives encourage ambulation (walking in labor) so they ask if that would be allowed for them. "Sure, we want to have you up and about...except for when we need to have you on the monitor, or of course, after you've had your pain relief."

"We won't be using pharmaceuticals." Mr. & Mrs. Anybody remind him.

"Huh?" He looks up from their chart. "Oh, right. Ok, if you say so." He says with a grin.

Midwives provide perineal support. Will he? "Of course," he says "unless I see that you really need an episiotomy, at which time I assume you want me to do one instead of letting you rip wide open."

"Certainly!" Mrs. Anyone agrees. He must make that determination. After all, that's why they hired him.

"We'd like the cord to stop pulsing before being cut." the parents request.

"Sure," The doctor amiably replies, "not a problem! Unless, of course, the baby needs to be resuscitated or you are hemorrhaging or something." He says in an off-hand manner as if it happens all the time.

"Of course." The parents say weakly, growing pale in the face as they picture these complications that must be so common that the doctor would mention them.

If 90% of communication is what is between the lines, these parents should be running, not walking, to the nearest exit. Instead, they tell themselves what a good thing it is they chose this doctor who will "let" them do what they want in labor. They have the 'best of both worlds' as far as they are concerned. They push down the feelings of unease that struggle to be acknowledged.

He tells them he is scheduling a triple test for next week, a gestational diabetes test for the week after, and an ultrasound for the week after that.

"We'd like to avoid further routine prenatal testing." The parents again must remind him.

"Of course you do!" he agrees. "I wouldn't suggest these if I didn't think they were important. You see, I'm concerned about your fundal height. The baby might not be growing as well as I'd like, so we need to have that ultrasound." (He doesn't add that repeated ultrasound is implicated in intra-uterine growth retardation—the condition he supposedly is looking for) (Wagner, 1999.)

He continues, "The triple test is probably not really necessary, but it's just a simple blood draw, no problem at all really. Not invasive. No reason not to do it if we can save you heartache down the road." (There is no mention of the fact this test has a high rate of false-positives that could result in immeasurable heartache) (Graves, Miller, & Sellers, 2002)

Adding, "Gestational diabetes is treatable. If you have it, wouldn't you want to know so that you could prevent the high rate of stillbirth that occurs with diabetic mothers?" (Again, no explanation that the high rate of still birth is with women who have a pre-existing condition or history of diabetes in the family, who may be

281

exhibiting signs or symptoms of manifesting the condition. Also no mention that the American Diabetes Association advises against routine testing of healthy women because there is no improvement in outcomes).* If you were my wife, I'd want you to have it."

He's been so cooperative, they go along with it. One test leads to another. He may even agree that some of the tests aren't necessary…unless. Somehow, there is always a reason, that seems legitimate, to have them done. Each ten-minute visit with Dr. So-and-so seems to build a relationship based on trust and full disclosure, yet they haven't really given true informed on anything. They may get their dream birth, but I wouldn't bet on it. Even if a couple has avoided the vast majority of unnecessary technology though pregnancy, the caregiver who misuses or overuses technology will find a way to justify his presence at the birth somehow by the time all is said and done.

You buy the ticket, you take the ride. As Nancy Wainer says "If you don't want surgery, don't go to a surgeon." It's not fair to the surgeon to expect him to practice midwifery. He's not a midwife. He's not trained in normalcy and he's not geared to sit around doing nothing until he's needed. The medical establishment is based on pathology. He's trained to do something…anything! Going to a hospital and hiring a doctor, but telling them "I'd like it to be as close to a home birth as possible" (something they hear all the time) is an unrealistic expectation.

*This was the recommendation at the time the first edition of Mother's Intention was released. With the worsening obesity epidemic, the 2012 recommendation of the ADA is that all women, even those not at risk, be tested, acknowledging that, "These new criteria will significantly increase the prevalence of GDM, primarily because only one abnormal value, not two, is sufficient to make the diagnosis. ADA recognizes the anticipated significant increase in the incidence of GDM diagnosed by these criteria and is sensitive to concerns about the "medicalization" of pregnancies previously categorized as normal." and further, "Admittedly, there are few data from randomized clinical trials regarding therapeutic interventions in women who will now be diagnosed with GDM…" ADA, (2012)

Remember, some doctors practicing in hospitals don't believe home birth is safe, despite all the contrary evidence that it is. If they did, they'd be doing them. You aren't going to change their belief system in the short time span of your pregnancy, so why would their behavior change? You have not altered their underlying assumptions about the very nature of birth and you won't because all around them they see 'evidence' to support their belief. Birth is a very scary event in the hospital. When I have done a string of hospital labor support jobs without home births to balance them out, I've started to doubt the safety of birth. I can't blame them if that's all they see. I agree…Yikes!

However, I take issue with the fact that those same people will avoid viewing several midwife-attended home births or reading any evidence that contradicts their paradigm. It may be true for them that birth is dangerous — perception is reality — but as a whole, it isn't supported by fact. It's very difficult for someone who has only operated from this fear base to just let you go happily about your birthing business.

To be insistent that you want all of the amenities of home to fit into the routines and schedules of the hospital and doctor is going to mean behind your back someone is going to be saying "If they want a home birth so bad, why don't they have one?" I've heard it…I'm not joking. Quite frankly, they have a point.

In some areas, freestanding birth centers fill the gap. The word FREESTANDING is vitally important here. If a birth center is contained within a hospital, or affiliated with a hospital or medical practice, it's most likely obstetrics as usual with pretty rooms and nice ladies.

Have you made out your birth plan? What are the details of your perfect birth? Take a moment, close your eyes, breathe deeply and imagine the perfect birth. Where did it take place? Who was there? Does this picture tell you anything about unconscious beliefs you didn't even know you held?

In composing your birth plan, what was important to you and why? How does your care provider feel about birth plans? Some online OB message boards are accessible to the general public...it makes for interesting reading about how they really feel. Some just dismiss them. Some are outright hostile to the idea. Some comment that a substantial birth plan is a sure cesarean. Would that be the fault of unrealistic expectations? Or, perhaps these couples are treated differently for expressing their wishes? Both, I believe. What might seem totally reasonable for a home or (freestanding) birthing center birth just doesn't translate well to an institution whose very existence is antithetical to the idea of natural birth.

Unfortunately, at this moment in history, we must pay very close attention to whether the words and actions of our health care representatives match. There are too many caregivers who have made it abundantly clear that they will not change—but they don't want to see that effect their pocketbook, so they say what they think you want to hear.

Admitting this ugly truth is cause for some caregivers to protest that advocates of safe and gentle birth are making parents distrustful of their caregivers. This again would be a classic case of shooting the messenger. This book would not exist if these things, sadly, didn't happen all over the country every day.

I am not fostering distrust. What I am encouraging is a healthy discernment. Parents have a right to verification of safety and efficacy. There are caregivers out there who practice more safely than current 'standard of care,' which, I will repeat, has been established not by medical evidence, but lawyers. As consumers ask more questions and demand better, more physicians will join those pioneering souls. Until that time, I'd wager that the good doctors would be willing to answer a few more questions than usual. The bad doctors don't even have to worry about going hungry...there are millions of women convinced that birth is something it isn't, not to mention the millions of women who don't want to put any effort into their health or their children, as evidenced by the child abuse, neglect and abandonment we see on the news daily. Remember, I'm not forcing anyone to have a great birth...I'm only guiding the ones who are willing to work for it.

Physicians have given consumers no other option. As long as bad doctors are allowed to abuse technology and poor outcomes on the whole are acceptable, parents can sue...or let their voices be heard through their wallets. Short of a whistle-blower lawsuit for the billions this out of control situation is costing the US government these are the only ways care will improve. If there is a shift in what parents are willing to accept, good doctors are rewarded. The others can choose to follow or not, but at least it won't be at the expense of you or your baby. It fosters accountability, not distrust. It's not expecting doctors to be something they aren't or hospitals to do the impossible by being 'just like home.' Hospitals are not home. They are places for the sick and injured, filled with highly skilled professionals, that must run efficiently to be effective.

You must decide what you really, truly want if you are going to be able to take steps to get it. You must be specific and you must ask yourself every step of the way if your decisions are based on fact.

Before now, you may not have thought you had a genuine chance of having a safe birth that was comfortable, too. For a very long time the desire to have a gentle birth has been placed in conflict with the desire for a safe birth (purposely, I might add, because the two are not mutually exclusive by any stretch of the imagination). Mothers have been asked, "Are you concerned about a 'good experience' or a live baby?" The two are very much interdependent!

Now that you know that, you may still be unsure about how to recognize and articulate exactly what it is you want. If all you've been offered is one of two options, how overwhelming to suddenly realize you can have it all if you want.

None-the-less, indecision creates inaction. Inertia leads, unintentionally, to birthing horror stories. Since you probably know exactly what you don't want, start where you are.

You don't need to limit this exercise to just your birth. Extend these ideas into early parenthood to give you a head start on what reality you are creating there.

You'll only get as much as you ask for and no more, so ask for the moon. If a series of events outside of your control alter what is possible, you are still striving for your own best ideal, but you need to identify what you want, make a plan for how you can make it happen and put the effort toward better birth. No one else will do this work for you. The world in general doesn't care if you have your ideal birth. Your childbirth educator shouldn't be working harder or putting more hours into your birth than you are. Your caregiver certainly won't put more time and effort into you birth than you. They shouldn't have to. It's your baby, your body, your life, your responsibility.

Having said that, be careful what you wish for. Your subconscious mind can take you very literally sometimes. If you keep telling yourself that all you want is a fast labor, you just may get a half hour birth that hits hard, fast, and furious.

You may think that's what you want, but mothers who are in the midst of a precipitous (very fast) labor don't know it's only going to last a half hour. Fear that the intensity could last indefinitely can engage the fear/tension/pain cycle, turning what might have been one painful contraction in a nearly painless birth into many in a painful one. If you still think your idea birth is fast, you may want to add 'comfortable' to your list of wants…and then plan to have your baby at home with a skilled caregiver so that you don't end up birthing in your car on the freeway with the help of a 911 operator.

Also, remember that this ideal birth you'd like to plan has a time limitation. You have nine months or less to optimize your health, choose a caregiver that will contribute to your experience without contaminating it, decide on birth location and become educated on the postpartum issues that round out what has been dubbed the 4th "trimester" of your childbearing year. Take the time to learn about the seemingly endless decisions you'll face after the birth. These can't wait until the last minute.

In order to avoid regret over any of these decisions, use the same tools you have learned in this book to create your birth. Many of these first decisions are often not made in conscious awareness. A great deal of myth and misconception surrounds each of the ones I've mentioned and I've only touched the tip of the iceberg.

The moments immediately following birth are primary. While it's true we don't bond with the first object we see like a gosling, the first interactions are vitally important to the developmental changes meant to occur within the mothers birthing brain and the baby's. (Klaus, Kennell, & Klaus, 1996) Neurological connections are being made now, including the number of new brain cells being produced through a complex mix of baby's first interactions, protection from chemical alteration and the presence of certain substances within the mother's milk.

Yes, mothers who are drugged during birth or who don't breastfeed love their babies. The bond is different, however. (Please note: I did not say 'less,' only different.) Mothers who have done it both ways attest to this. We aren't being honest with ourselves if we insist that disruptions to the natural mammalian bonding mechanism don't have any effect at all. Narcotics in labor are still narcotics. If they impact your baby while you are pregnant, they impact your baby in labor. Artificial baby formula is not just a replacement food for babies; it circumvents the flood of hormones though out the mother, particularly oxytocin and prolactin, that are meant to create a visceral bonding experience. To insist that the experiences are exactly the same, when all of the elements right down to a chemical level are different, is disingenuous.

The irony is, some of the mothers who would say this are the same ones who complain that it took them months to fall in love with their baby and that this bonding thing is all a farce in the very next breath. They'd rather blame nature than admit they started out at with a deficit they must compensate for. If they haven't done it another way, they can't possibly know if there is a difference, which mothers who have insist there is. Science says there's a difference. Biology is not an opinion. Nature provided us with the same chemicals and instincts for the protection of our offspring as were provided to other mammals. (Odent, 1999) Other mammals will reject their offspring, refuse to protect them, even attack them, if the first moments of birth are disrupted and nursing of babies is prevented.

Baby's first days, weeks and months lay the foundation for how they will learn, how they relate to the world, how big their brains will be, what disease they will be susceptible to and even how fat or thin they will be as adults. (Carr-Morse & Wiley, 1997) These are not things to be taken lightly or to worry about later.

There is a window of opportunity, from birth to three years, that never, ever opens again. (Pearce,1992; Liedloff, 1995; Blaffer Hrdy, 1999) It would be devastating to learn the ramification of careless choices too late. This requires prioritizing. You must discover what's meaningful and important—with foresight, not in hindsight.

· What do you want for your child? For yourself? Not in vague terms like but very specifically, what are the specific components to what you consider ideal. It sounds like a simple question, but to one person happiness is security, while another is adventure. A 155 pound four year-old didn't suddenly expand when he turned four. Certainly, what the child eats as a four year-old and the amount of movement he engages in supports his overweight condition, there is no doubt. The anguish the mother of this child feels and the health problems this child faces very likely has its roots in the very first substance that child was given...either sugar water or formula. Does that mean that infants fed artificial baby milk will be fat adults? It depends on if the rest of their life contributes to the original damage or not. It depends on genetics. It depends on a lot of things, but giving our infants nothing but the equivalent of baby junk-food through the most highly formative period of their life ensures they have three strikes against them.

· How do you get to where you want to be? If happiness for you is a close knit, loving family, sitting around the fire playing games on family game night, you must build that brick by brick. Do you think you will have a close relationship if your child has spent 80% of their waking hours being parented by a parental substitution?

· If you had your ideal, how does it differ from now? How can you make it happen? Are your proposed parenting choices propelling or impeding your efforts?

If you can't answer these questions right this minute, you have serious work to do. Your birth is not something you can plan to coast through, parenthood even less so.

It's ok to admit you want this once in a lifetime event to be peaceful, comfortable and empowering. 'Safe' fits into all of those. If you have one of those exceedingly rare complications of pregnancy, your field of possibilities may narrow, but it should not be obliterated.

Keep in mind that many variations of normal are now used as excuses to cut babies out, even when outcomes haven't improved with the effort. If you want to keep your vision of a better birth in mind, you have to know the difference between a variation and a true complication. You have to know if something like a malpresentation is preventable, fixable or workable. You need to be willing to get a second opinion on subjective things like 'too big' of a baby, 'too small' of a pelvis, 'too much' water, 'too little' water. You must be knowledgeable about things like fundal height so that if you are told it's too high or too low you know what simple things, such as the baby's position, can affect it.

You need to be aware (and believe!) that being pregnant 42 weeks is perfectly fine as long as you and the baby are healthy and that there are non-invasive ways to assess fetal well-being.

Don't depend on luck when it comes to your life or that of your baby's. Knowing why you want something is as important as knowing what you want. 'I want a natural birth' can mean you want your baby's brain free from chemicals that may alter his brain structure. It may mean you want to feel the strength, pride and sense of accomplishment a natural labor rewards one with. It could just mean you are afraid of surgery. Move toward something you want, instead of running away from what you don't.

To some women 'natural' encompasses, albeit by stretching the limits of the English language, any tool that keeps them comfortable, while other women—believe it or not—would rather feel pain. There are payoffs for all of these women for the experience they choose.

The following conversation has taken place with countless variables. Twins, breech, cesarean, induction, you name it. I'll use VBAC for this example because cesareans have continued to rise for years.

Childbirth Educator (CBE): In considering your birth preferences, have you decided what's important to you for this birth?
Parent: I want a vaginal birth, if at all possible. Recovery was very hard after my section and I didn't feel really bonded with my baby for nearly a year. I got depressed and everything.
CBE: What efforts have you made toward that goal?
Parent: Well, I've talked to my doctor about it and he encourages it, as long as nothing goes wrong. I'm just not sure I should get my hopes up. I mean, my OB is really nice and all. He wants this for me as much as I do. But, the cesarean for my last child was because the induction didn't work, and my doctor says if I go past my due date, he'll have to induce me, or if the baby gets to big, he'll induce. It's hospital policy that if I don't go into labor during daylight hours

while the anesthesiologist is there, or if I'm in labor but it doesn't look like I'll deliver before he goes home, that they will just do the cesarean.

CBE: How would you feel if this birth were to be similar to your last birth?

Parent: I just couldn't stand it! If I get that depressed again I'm going to ask for an anti-depressant, even if it means I have to stop breastfeeding, if I even can breastfeed. It was so hard before. But, I'd deal with it, you know. You have to. You just wonder if there was something you could have done different. You know, disappointed, but you have to do what's best for the baby. That's all that matters...a healthy baby.

CBE: So what you really want is what is safest for you and the baby, preferably emotionally satisfying as well?

Parent: Yeah. I'm just afraid I won't meet all of the conditions that my doctor feels are important for our safety.

CBE: Would those be the conditions you just mentioned?

Parent: Yes. Plus, he says I have to have an epidural because if there is an emergency, they don't want to have to wait to place one. And, of course we have to have continuous electronic fetal monitoring in case of uterine rupture.

CBE: So what do you know about each of those interventions and their affect on labor? What would have to happen for you to be able to avoid those interventions that are known to increase surgical deliveries without any demonstrable benefits to outcomes with their use?

Parent: I don't know. I guess I don't have a choice. My doctor won't do it without all of these conditions. I think it's hospital policy or something. (sounding distraught) See! I knew I couldn't do it.

CBE: Why would you feel a sense of failure on your part? Are these conditions in your best interest and based on fact? Do you have control over any of these conditions?

Parent: (perplexed) I don't know. I guess I don't have much control, if any, over them. But they must have these rules for a reason. I know my doctor wouldn't do it if he didn't have to. I mean, he's helped a lot of women have VBACs, so they must be Ok.

CBE: What percentage of his VABC mothers actually have vaginal births?

Parent: (sounding angry) I don't know! A lot, I'm sure. He's a very good doctor! What do you think I should do?

CBE: You have hard decisions to make. I can help you access the information you need to make evidence-based decisions, but you have to do the work and make the hard choices.

Parent: Do you think my doctor is a bad doctor? (sounding defensive)

CBE: My job is to help parents make their own best decisions using the latest scientific literature available. I don't know your doctor. I only know what the evidence says. In order to help you clarify if you are on the path to have the birth you say you want, why don't you tell me how you would feel if your dream of a natural birth were realized?

Parent: Proud of myself. Happy. Strong. Capable. I assume physically better. Glad that I did the best I could.

CBE: So, You'd like to feel whole, proud, fulfilled, strong and empowered?

Parent: Yes! Then I could connect with my baby better. Maybe I could feel like I didn't fail as a woman and I could concentrate on being a mother instead of dealing with depression and healing from surgery.

CBE: What do you need to do to maximize the possibility of that outcome?

Parent: If it's going to happen, I guess it's up to me. I'll look into those interventions my doctor insists on, and if they aren't in our best interest and based on fact, I won't agree to them. I hope I don't have to, but if he won't work with us, I'll change doctors and find someone who will.

In reality, conversations like this have usually ended at, "I don't know...what do you think I should do?" because the CBE won't take responsibility for the birth. It wouldn't matter if the CBE gave her a point by point strategic disassemble of everything that was wrong with the illogic behind that conversation and a bulleted list of what the mom could do to change it...she still wouldn't do it. I know. I've tried! Silly me, I thought when I was asked for advice I was actually supposed to give it and the people who asked actually asked because they wanted to follow it!

Women know down in their heart what's right. It is their mother's intuition and it guides them well…if they would only listen.

Listen to your heart and the small voice within. Don't be deterred from what you know is best for you and your baby.

There are, unfortunately, people out there who have a stake in what you think, feel and believe about birth and early parenting. Your thoughts control their bottom line. That is honesty, not pessimism.

If you have the strength and resolve to believe you deserve to get a gentle, safe birth, you make possible what others see as impossible. If you make your choices based on fact and stick to your decisions, the improbable becomes probable. Then, even if your birth falls short of your ideal, you can be free of guilt or regret. You will know you have done everything in your power to create your own best birth.

If you've never demand better for yourself, it may feel odd to demand better for yourself and your baby. Consider it your first act of motherhood…protecting your young, ensuring that your baby has only the very best.

Consider if you were able to hand pick the parent who would raise your child if you couldn't. What qualities, characteristics and behaviors would you expect? Would it be good enough to just keep the kid alive, or would you expect interaction that would nurture body, mind, and soul? Would minimum contact be enough, or would you want loving contact? Is impatient, distracted communication enough, or would you want respectful, meaningful exchanges?

Do you meet the criteria you would expect of another? Resolve now to do what it takes to ensure the emotional, spiritual and physical best for your child. It may inconvenience some people who might be irritated that you won't 'just do what everyone else does.' How many of those people love that precious little being growing inside you as much as you do?

Is your sweet baby worth a little extra effort? A little bit of sacrifice? Is your baby worth going the extra mile? How many opportunities do you think you get to impact the world through direct action? It's a wonderful life. Make it count.

CHAPTER 14

Dream It, Do It

By now, I hope you've become convinced that birth can be anything from orgasmic to manageably sufferable and everything in between.

Most of what we experience arises directly from those beliefs and expectations about birth from which we make our decisions. A small percentage of undesirable outcomes result naturally, but far more are happening that are preventable.

The variables are endless, the experience subjective. The promise of this book is that you can create better birth—better than what our culture at large is experiencing, better than what you would create if all of your actions were dictated by unconscious motivations stemming from faulty core assumptions.

It assumes no choice inherently right or wrong in every situation, only that purity of intent be the assessment tool by which an action is measured. It passes no judgment on a particular caregiver, action or birth location…only on unsubstantiated claims of safety and efficacy.

Knowledge is power…knowledge of the system, knowledge of the process, knowledge of your self. When I teach a childbirth class, I begin with the question "How much of the childbirth and parenting information you feel you need do you expect to be provided from this class?" The response is often 75-100%! This is a totally unrealistic expectation! With an eight-hour investment of their time, they expect to learn what should actually take at least a year! In compiling this book I had to set aside enough information for space considerations that a whole separate book was born to be a companion to this one.

I do not claim to have all of the answers. I do not expect anyone to substitute my considered opinion for their own convictions. I do expect them to become aware of whether or not those assumptions are based on fact or fiction and are in the best interest of their baby.

I am confident you can create your own best birth. I encourage you to explore the recommended reading and independent childbirth classes. Some sources are better than others. If a source has a vested interest in influencing your choices, it should be deemed secondary to independent sources. This is an organizational conflict of interest, yet this is the source parent's have singularly depended on for years.

Throughout this book you have eliminated inconsistencies in what you believe you can achieve and what you want to have. You know what is clearly within your control. You know that what you experience in the first few months as a mother is directly related to what you experience in birth. In order to attain the highest success for yourself in birth, you need to assess where you stand.

If there is still a wiggly feeling that resembles guilt, ask yourself if you are being brutally honest with yourself about whether it's a matter of 'can't' or 'won't.' No one is judging you during this exercise. No one can see what's in your heart but you. If your mother's intuition is telling you something, it's a private communication to you and you alone.

If you are doing the best you can with what you have, know that's all any of us can do. Do not compare yourself with anyone else. Rather, use your perception of others to try to get an idea of how reasonable you are being about your situation.

Remember that often what we think is true about others is only an illusion. All that matters is your own intent; your own motivation; your own assessment of what you are capable of. That inner voice may not be guilt…it may be sadness that you cannot provide what you feel best. Or, it might be guilt. Is it justified? Do you have options that bring you closer to your ideal, but you aren't choosing them because you are confusing a want with a need? Is this discrepancy something you can live with, or will it tear you apart with every reminder that you didn't rise to your own potential for the sake of your child? People have achieved greatness against seemingly impossible odds. A parent who wants to excel at parenthood is certainly capable if they make it a priority.

Once it's clear where the discrepancies are, you have the choice of reassessing how what you say and what you do mesh, or you can realign your investment to reflect your priorities.

Preparing--bringing your priorities and your attention together.

Prenatally, this can be put to work by making a birth plan and then ensuring that your actions bring about optimal results. It's imperative to lay the groundwork for your birth preferences early. A caregiver cannot honor your birth plan if you have set up conditions that require the use of the things you say you don't want. Use a multitude of resources to construct your birth plan. You can learn about your options through a number of places, including the internet, books, and classes.

· Keep it short. Midwives, doctors and nurses are very busy and often won't even have a chance to get through anything over a page or two.
· Be polite. This isn't a list of demands, it's the ideal picture you have in mind for your birth. It is a gateway to respectful communication. Request nicely and make sure you thank your birth team in advance for their help in creating this ideal.
· Be clear that you are flexible. Again, this is your wish list for your birth, but it's important that you let your care providers know that in the case of true medical indication, you are certainly willing to alter it. You have the right (and responsibility) to understand the rationale for any intervention you agree to...this is called informed consent and it is for the protection of both you and your provider. You may ask about the perceived problem, why it is a problem, what the treatment might be, what the side effects are and if there are

alternatives. In the event of a time sensitive emergency, you may get an abbreviated reply, so it is wise to be familiar with possible interventions and the medical indications beforehand. The Thinking Woman's Guide to Better Birth by Henci Goer is a good resource.

· Be clear in your reasoning. You don't have to fill your birth plan with medical journal abstracts, but be prepared to back up your choices with language Your providers are familiar with. They have little patience for people who want to go against protocol 'just because.' Let them know that there are solid reasons behind your choices, that you choices are safe and that they are supported by evidence. Henci Goer has compiled just such a resource in a book with scientific evidence from medical journals called Obstetric Myths versus Research Realities that can help you.

· Use Positive Language. Fill the plan with what you do prefer, not what you don't want. By keeping the tone of your birth plan positive, respectful and reasonable, you will very likely be able to create a unified birth team and have a safe and satisfying birth experience.

Create your perfect birth visualization remembering it's important to make sure that it contains the elements required to elicit the relaxation response discussed previously. What does it smell like? Feel like? Sound like? Who is there? What time of day is it? What time of year? If you have set up your environment to support and maintain the relaxation response throughout a normal, natural birth, it's quite possible that a painless birth, or at least relatively comfortable birth, may be expected. However, it's important to understand that going it alone will probably be less effective than using a program that has worked for thousands of women.

This birth belongs to you alone. The events of your birth-day will rest in your heart...either sustaining or haunting. You are accountable only to your own heart...and to your child.

Putting it all together

You've done great work! You should now have a plan for safe birth in mind and the courage to implement it. Let's get specific about how to put it into action.

First, define your idea of a great birth in behavioral terms. Not "All I want is a healthy baby", but how you plan to create a foundation of wellness that optimize the health of your baby. What are the very real, concrete steps to this end? What do you have to eat? What might you have to change in your life in the way of stress or work or exercise?

If your better birth were just a wish, it would be all right to be vague. "I want a natural birth" is wide open to interpretation. If you want it to happen, it's necessary to paint a picture for your subconscious mind and use enough detail so that you can clearly establish what steps are required to reach it.

For instance, does "I want a natural birth" mean you want a drug free birth? A painless birth? Does it mean you are only willing to commit to draw on your own reserves for a set amount of time before you allow yourself to make a determination that you are willing to ask for drugs? You'll need to define your objective and then figure out how it can best be accomplished. What will you need to do...or not do? How will you know it's happening the way you want before, during, and after? What is the emotional impact of doing your birth your way?

Next, decide you will evaluate your progress in realizing your dream birth. In the above example, to have your natural birth, where would you have to plan to give birth? Who would you allow at your birth? Which caregiver? Would you have a doula? Is your partner contributing positively to your effort? What needs to be done to get everyone on the same page? What comfort measures will you stock your 'bag of tricks' with?

How do you think you'll behave your way to your own best birth? How much time do you need to devote to this ideal every single day to make it happen? Create a schedule for yourself in which you can take 'baby steps'.

Idea:

Purchase some beautiful beads and a necklace that allows you to add and remove beads easily. Use one bead to represent each week of your pregnancy that remains in order to give you a visual reminder of the importance of taking immediate steps to reach your pregnancy goals. For example, say you are 12 weeks along...you will have 30 beads. 42 weeks (remembering that 40 weeks is merely an average and that 42 weeks is perfectly normal) minus the 12 weeks that have already passed leave you with potentially 30 week. Thus 30 beads in your necklace. As you remove a bead from your string each week, it gives you something visual of how much time remains in which to make adjustments to your plan. You may even map out what you need to do, week by week, and chart your progress in a journal as you removed a bead from your necklace each week.

Approach each week as a celebration, with tangible efforts and rewards for being a part of the procreative process. Each week make a promise to take three actions that would be required to achieve your perfect birth. Use a body, mind, spirit approach. What can you physically do to increase the odds of a natural birth? Stop smoking? Exercise? Visit a nutritionist? Take a pregnancy yoga class?

What can you do to educate yourself? Take a class? Read a book per week? Think about your birth plan and create an outline?

Remember your spirit...honor your role as a co-creator in this most sacred task of creating a human being. You may want to visit a certified hypnotherapist to clear away any trauma from your own birth or a past birth. You may want to journal, forgive a parent or explore your special connection with the Divine through art. Write it down, manifest your reality.

If you have five different bead colors, use them to create a repeating pattern, then use corresponding colors of markers or pens to write down what you promise to do on each week you remove another bead.

In order to avoid getting discouraged, map out only what you control and remain flexible. You control the state of your health (in large measure), your emotions, who you hire or fire in your maternity care, where you will plan to give birth. You cannot control the actions of others (though you have complete control over what you will put up with), you cannot control the weather and in very rare instances, nature will throw you a curve for which you will have to alter your plans. If this happens, it does not mean all is lost! It means this is your first of many lessons in patience and adaptability that comes with being a parent.

Flexibility requires a good working knowledge of your possible obstacles and resources. Take a proactive approach to dealing with any hindrances that might occur. Set up your environment to support your efforts. Make "Because I'm the mommy, that's why!" your mantra!

Be gentle with yourself, but not permissive. Don't take a guilt trip if you don't meet a goal one week...but also don't allow breaking promises to yourself, your baby and your partner become a habit. Feel good about doing your best as long as you are making progress. Take charge of what you have control over and accept that which you don't.

This is a good place to pull your partner in to help you stay true to yourself. Be sure to communicate clearly that what you need is a sympathetic team player...not a warden or baby sitter. If you know someone is keeping tabs on your efforts, you are more likely to self-monitor. However, you don't need someone following you around with a notebook recording each bite you take, stocking the pantry goodies you are trying to avoid, or telling you to get more sleep, then demanding to know why his underwear hasn't been washed!

Taking these last steps may be leaving you feeling empowered, but overwhelmed. Excited, but anxious. It's liberating to know that your options are more plentiful than you imagined, but scary that there are so many choices. Knowing that you are the determining factor in the sort of birth you create can be terrifying as well as exhilarating.

Work with the facts. You are not being asked to substitute anyone else's ideas, observations or beliefs for your own. I would never expect anyone to agree with me 100%. We all know what we know (or think we know) based on the information we've been exposed to (or sought out) and our particular life experiences. I'm not in your shoes. All I can do is share the information, which is neutral in and of itself. If you don't agree with the data, it may not seem neutral to you, but apply the standards set forth in previous chapters to test validity.

Only by examining your beliefs — and questioning mine — will you be able to decide if you are part of the silent and exceedingly sad epidemic of birthing apathy that has resulting in unacceptable national statistics and troubling social tribulations.

Midwives often say we birth as we live. I say, it also works the other way. All areas of our life, beginning with our issues of self-worth, are affected by how we give birth.

You may still choose trial and error methods, hoping that you have a nice birth and accepting the penalty for not being fully engaged. That's your prerogative. I believe in mothers. I think they will rise to their calling if they know they do matter. Devaluing a mother's contribution has left us with a collective despondency that has left mothers with little direction.

I believe that as we lift ourselves up, we gain momentum. Eventually, as we expect more of ourselves, feeling the joy and deep, deep feelings of love and devotion our biology has provided us with to care for our babies, we will reach a point of critical mass.

The positive and far-reaching implications will generate changes in our lives that will transform our communities, our country and our world.

You now have the awareness, knowledge and clarity to make a fairytale birth your reality. What you do with it is up to you. You can learn from the mistakes of sad, angry, and frustrated mothers, or repeat them. You can begin to see synchronicity and grace or ignore it. You can decide to focus on the positive, or let the negative drag you down. Ignoring the negative only makes you susceptible to it.

If you let people intimidate or manipulate you into disregarding your mother's intuition, the valuable insights this book could provide are lost. Live your own best life, create your own best birth, love your baby before all else. That is all that is important in this life.

If what you've been doing isn't working, change it. If what you are being told doesn't make sense, challenge it. Reject it if it isn't based on fact or not in your best interest. Policies that help your doctor or a hospital avoid malpractice are not your concern. If protocol and procedure is not for the benefit of you and your baby, why submit to it?

Why be cheated out of video of your baby's first moments because someone has a fear of litigation...these are your baby's first moments, never to happen ever again! Condition yourself to question those motivations...where is the concern that the doctor might have reason to fear litigation? Why is it when the hospital tour includes expensive and elaborate security measures, including lock down and baby tagging, parents are in awe, instead of being alarmed that such measures would be necessary?

Choose a positive attitude and healthy behaviors to optimize your birth outcome. Study the successes and failures as you perceive them around you. Emulate the successes. Refuse to repeat failure...as you see it. Seek support for a gold-standard birth because how we birth does matter. Believe all things are possible.

Of course there is no actual 'right' or 'wrong', no 'success' or 'failure' other than your own perception. By success I mean emulating that which is beneficial to you, body, mind and soul. By 'failure' I mean that which harms. I'm not implying you should try to be someone you aren't....only the best you can be.

I am saying that if you look around you will find women who have had joyful, ecstatic or orgasmic and painless births that can be role models if that is the experience you desire.

There are parents that seem 'lucky' because their children are calm, peaceful, smarter than 'average' or hardly ever sick. It isn't an accident and it isn't luck. We know what parenting skills produce those results in uncompromised children. It isn't that luck never enters into the equation, but there is a demonstrable cause and affect relationship to nearly every childhood development or behavior.

What is it those parents are doing? It's worth your time to scrutinize and evaluate their strategies. Do you admire their philosophies? Is there an underlying philosophy that their success hinges on? Do you share that attitude or can you adopt it? Do they have a strong commitment and ethics that you respect? Will they take risks to put their children first? Do your children have the same types of personalities as theirs?

Most likely, they share certain parental characteristics that make the difference between exceptional parenting and parenting by default. They have a firm conceptualization of what it means (to them) to be a good parent and what actions they need to take to be that. They aren't afraid of doing what it takes for the sake of their children's well-being.

These parents are sure of what's right for their children and why. They don't care what other parents do because they know that only they live with the consequences of their actions. They are informed before making decisions, so there is no regret or guilt...only learning.

They allow their children to unfold at their own pace, developing their own individuality.

Exceptional parents are passionate about what they do. They know there is no job more important than raising children. They don't just give parenthood lip service. They make a real investment of themselves. They hold themselves to high standards and speak their truth. They feel no need to defend their actions and value any and all information that might help them grow as parents. They understand the demands required to do a job well and accept them.

They meet challenges with flexibility, accepting input on all viable alternatives and reserve the right to change their minds at any time if new information comes along...and do so without apology for doing the best they can with what they have.

Great parents are willing to face the unknown as an adventure instead of a threat. They are willing to grow. Their maxim is 'Change is inevitable, growth is optional.' They do not see themselves as the shapers of young minds as much as co-learners. They respect their children from the beginning and demand that others treat their children with respect. They honor what their children can teach them.

Strong ties and deep bonding are important in these families. They like being together. The parents enjoy their children's company, and value the need for their time as a couple as well as alone time. They orchestrate balance in their lives.

Effective parenting demands that priorities are set and that self-management ensures priorities are kept. They keep promises to themselves and their children from day one. They make sure their actions match their words...because children understand to their core that people show you who they are. Children internalize what you do, not what you say. Their concepts of self-worth are built on where they fall on your priority list, and their level of self-esteem determines who they become. Yes, they are born with certain aptitudes, but what they will do with them is shaped solely on whether you nurture or corrupt their gifts.

You make a difference! Do not trivialize your contribution to the whole, or allow anyone else to do so. Take pride in how you approach this special role you've accepted. It's a gift.

Every choice, every thought, every action, every moment of every day, makes you the parent you are. You are the only mother (or father) your child will ever have. The baby within you is enveloped physically, energetically, emotionally in what you are. You are building the body and brain that will be home to your child's soul for a lifetime. You get one chance. You are unique. Only you know what is right for you and what is acceptable or preferable for you and your baby. I hope by now you realize that you have special license to be outspoken, non-conformist, and certainly even a little demanding. You are the only one who can speak for your baby, protect your baby, and make life decisions for your baby. Decide that you have a special entitlement as a mother holding generations within you. As long as what you want or need is in accordance with free will and for the good for of all, not at the expense of others, you have a right to it. Remember, intention makes the difference.

(Almost) The Last Word

Throughout this work I have repeatedly referred to 'evidence-based care.' Yet, the book itself is called Mother's Intention. It may seem that there is a dichotomy here in placing the focus on a mother's intentions when much of the problem isn't that mothers aren't well intentioned, but that they aren't being offered evidence-based options. But there is no contradiction. Change will not happen if it doesn't begin with us...women, mothers, consumers.

The reason I have insisted on testing the validity of facts is due to the current hypocrisy in which medical authorities dissuade the use of integrative therapies, herbal remedies or natural options because 'they aren't approved by the FDA' or 'haven't been studied,' yet so

306

many of the drugs used in obstetrics have not been studied and are not approved.

This same hypocrisy allows doctors to discount traditional midwives or childbirth educators as autonomous practitioners because they don't have a degree, thus, the claim is, their care or advice is not predicated on science...yet admittedly the majority of what is considered 'standard of care' in obstetrics today is disproved by this science they claim so essential. No science is better than bad science.

The Hippocratic Oath, supposed to be a promise to serve, reads in part:

> I will apply, for the benefit of the sick, all measures which are required, avoiding those twin traps of over-treatment and therapeutic nihilism. I will remember that there is art to medicine as well as science, and that warmth, sympathy, and understanding may outweigh the surgeon's knife or the chemist's drug. My responsibility includes these related problems, if I am to care adequately for he sick.
>
> Louis Lasagna, Academic Dean of the School of Medicine, Tufts University 1964 (Tyson, 2001)

Dr. David Graham in JAMA, the Journal of the American Medical Association December 2000 issue states:

> "The original oath is redolent [evocative, reminiscent] of a covenant, a solemn and binding treaty." (ibid.)

Nearly 100 percent of graduating doctors pledge this promise of harming none...so how can what is happening to birthing women continue?

This oath is supposed to be our promise that if we surrender ourselves to the physician in our most weak and vulnerable of times, our health and well-being will come before personal profit, establishments, ego or HMO.

Who will require more of these who would take such an oath so casually? It's up to us. We must require more of ourselves so that others will be lifted to their own best self. We must do it for the babies. We must honor those who have not lost site of the greater good.

We have the best resources in the developed world. We can be one of the safest places on the planet to birth. We can make it happen.

Afterword

Writing a book is often compared to having a baby. It's a fair comparison.

It takes longer to write a book...and get it published. Having a baby was easier (in my humble opinion) although both processes are gratifying, as is the sense of accomplishment at the end-result.

During the writing of *Mother's Intention*, birthing stories crossed my desk continually. It would be hard to explain the feelings that surfaced as I saw such vivid examples of what happens when unconscious fear dictates action. I would wonder, with great curiosity, how so many mothers whose conscious impetus was safe birth, would insist that there was no time to take a childbirth class, yet frenetically try to 'tie things up' at work or get the baby's room finished. What could cause a caring mother to make unwise choices, resist information that would help her make safer decisions, and prioritize insignificant and trivial concerns above the baby's birth?

As you've already learned, there is a pay-off for our actions or we wouldn't do what we do. I wondered if all the busy work and avoidance of real issues was a distraction tactic. I marveled that, in many cases, it's not just a matter of avoiding exposure to anything that might contradict a belief, but actively putting a considerable amount of energy into avoiding it!

We've explored why parents do such things in great depth throughout this work. By the time I got to the end I began to wonder how many other factors are involved in the millions of women who are willing to settle so cheap and make motherhood so much harder.

What else could make women choose what they are choosing? Other works have explored anthropological and sociological factors. I've heard theories that there could be women who make the experience as hard as possible to prove a point…either to prove they can endure such an ordeal, or to 'prove' joyful birth proponents wrong.

I would venture a guess that there are many women who have such low self-esteem that they feel they don't deserve a wonderful birth, and others who have such low expectations of themselves that they don't want to consider that birth can be amazing, lest they be unable to attain such a 'lofty' ideal. Maybe such a woman would be so insecure that the fear of not being able to 'do it' means they would just rather not even try.

It seems to me, fear and false birth beliefs are still at the root, but what keeps these beliefs alive?

They are actively fed. Consider the example of artificial induction of labor mentioned throughout Mother's Intention and the cavalier attitude about it that sabotages an enormous number of parents with the best intent.

Say a woman goes in for a prenatal visit near the end of the pregnancy and during the visit she is given her routine (worthless and dangerous) internal exam, which may seem unusually uncomfortable. She may or may not be aware of what has happened, but her care provider has just 'striped her membranes'…inserted a finger through the opening of the cervix and run it around the circumference of the cervix to initiate labor.

(She also may not know he has a golf outing planned for the weekend--or a New Year's party, or a vacation scheduled--and wants to get this labor started so she won't have her baby while he's away.)

Parents may question the wisdom of rushing nature for convenience, but are often told, "Sure, there could be a small amount of risk…as there is in anything…but we do this all the time and rarely encounter problems."

If she has agreed to the procedure, this mom probably was not told that it could likely result in premature rupture of her membranes, or that it increases her chance of infection. Neither would she probably be told that if she fails to go into labor after the water breaks, she will be on a clock to deliver within 12 hours because her caregiver would be concerned about...are you ready for this...infection. The next step after this seemingly innocuous intervention is probably going to be one of two drugs, neither of which is approved by the FDA for elective labor induction.

So, in the next day or two, her water might break, and she may have surges...or she may not. But she will definitely now be in the hospital, with fingers in her often to assess her (slow) progress. Of course it's 'slow'...she probably wasn't quite ready. Even if she was, it will seem 'slow' to her caregiver, because now he's got to wrap this up before his engagement (and that threat of infection...that wasn't there until he put it there).

As he suggests cytotec or pitocin, he will downplay the risk because he wants her compliant. He may or may not give an actual risk factor to the intervention except to say that it's 'small.' He's probably right. The odds may be in his favor that nothing bad will happen.

What he fails to explain is what the odds are that this intervention will lead to another, which could lead to any number of serious problems, and ultimately unnecessary surgery. Nor will he be pointing out that although the risk for this particular intervention is low, the rate of complications associated with this cascade of interventions was ZERO before he purposely injected them into the situation. Or, that even if she avoids surgery, pitocin may turn her labor into a nightmare from which she begs to be rescued.

How many parents buy what he's selling? Probably most. The caregiver is banking on the fact that the odds he's playing with your baby's life are in his favor, and he's right. Sort of.

Moving ahead to the probable conclusion of a safe delivery, let's imagine (it appears) we have a healthy mom and baby. Everyone is happy that it all turned out, and the belief that concern was unjustified is reinforced. Mom and baby need to stay in the hospital a few days, instead of being able to go right home (which is probably where they would have been better off all along), exposing them both to a hospital-acquired infection.

At home, the baby is unresponsive to normal stimuli. "What a good baby!" everyone exclaims. The baby may not be interested in nursing, either because the jaundice from the pitocin makes him sleepy, or because of the narcotics, starting a vicious cycle ending with inadvertent weaning and much frustration. Mothers don't then blame the system that created this issue. Mothers blame themselves.

These problems could have been avoided, but since they weren't, they need to be managed without causing more damage. They can be overcome, it's just going to take a lot of effort to make it work.

In our culture, mothers are encouraged to be content with this. It's a 'good birth', if the mother and baby survive; bonus if they do it without getting cut. Even though the ecstasy of birth and deep bonding have been lost, if the parents are happy with what they have, that's good enough. I do support the right of mothers to have the birth they want…as long as it's not to the detriment of the baby…I just find it incredibly sad that 'good enough' is all they wish for themselves.

Deep down on a soul level I think we know when we've been robbed of our bliss…or we've voluntarily given it away. I can't imagine a bigger disservice to women than letting them think that's all there is!

When all is said and done, the parents are so glad that they got to have their baby before their doctor left town instead of having his back up, who is known to be quick with the knife.

Why is there such gratitude that their caregiver cared so little about them that he was willing to leave them in the hands of a colleague he's reasonably sure would subject mother and baby to an unnecessary major abdominal surgery? And, who was so self-absorbed that instead of putting the one and only birth of their baby first, was willing to introduce a number of potentially very harmful interventions to ensure he wouldn't miss a minute of his own plans. Why isn't this questioned? It's a blatant disregard of the 'do no harm' oath!

What if the other probable outcome happened, instead of this 'good' one? What if the interventions lead to a surgical birth as so many of them do?

Still, 'As long as everyone's ok now…that's all that matters' is what we've been conditioned to say, in order to not make the mother feel what, by now, you know we can't make a mother feel. Why (Oh, why?!) doesn't anyone question this line of reasoning? Just because what's been broken can (probably) be fixed does not mean it's ok to break it on purpose! Can you think of any other service or industry in which that might be okay?

Essentially, women's feelings are devalued by this type of comment hundreds of times a day. Most of those mothers are women who avoided the information you've just read with a 'see no evil' attitude, thinking nothing bad could happen to them if they just closed their eyes to reality. Please, don't be one of them.

Selected Bibliography

Baldwin, R., (1986). *Special Delivery: A Guide to Creating the Birth You Want for You and Your Baby*, Celestial Arts.

Benson, H., (2000). *The Relaxation Response*, revised ed., Harper Torch.

Benson, H., (1985). *Beyond the Relaxation Response*, Berkley Books.

Blaffer Hrdy, S., (1999). *Mother Nature; A History of Mothers, Infants and Natural Selection*, Pantheon Books.

Brookfield, S., (1991). *Developing Critical Thinkers: Challenging Adults to Explore Alternative Ways of Thinking and Acting*, Jossey-Bass.

Brookfield, S., (1995). *Becoming a Critically Reflective Teacher,* Jossey-Bass.

Cohen & Estner, (1983). *Silent Knife: Vaginal Birth After Cesarean and Cesarean Prevention*, Bergen and Garvey.

Cohen, N., (2000). *Open Season: A Survival Guide for Natural Childbirth and VBAC in the 90s*, Praeger Trade.

Dilts, (1990). *Changing Belief Systems with NLP*, Meta Publications.

England & Horowitz, (1998). *Birthing from Within*, Partera Press.

Enkin, Keirse, Renfrew & Neilson, (1995). *A Guide to Effective Care in Pregnancy and Childbirth*, 2nd Ed., Oxford University Press.

Frye, A., (1993). *Understanding Diagnostic Tests in the Childbearing Year, A Guide for Givers and Receivers of Health Care in Childbearing*, 5th ed., Labrys Press.

Frye, A., (1995). *Holistic Midwifery: A Comprehensive Textbook for Midwives in Homebirth Practice*, Vol, 1, Labrys Press.

Gaskin, I., (2003). *Ina May's Guide to Childbirth,* Bantam-Doubleday-Dell.

Gilovich, T., (1991). *How We Know What Isn't So: The Fallibility of Human Reason in Everyday Life*, The Free Press.

Goer, H., (1995). *Obstetric Myths versus Research Realities: A Guide to the Medical Literature*, Bergin and Garvey.

Goer, H., (1999). *The Thinking Woman's Guide to a Better Birth*, Perigree.

Gopnik, Meltzoff, Kuhl, (1999). *The Scientist in the Crib: Minds, Brains and How Children Learn*, William Morrow and Co.

Gordon, T., (2000). *Parent Effectiveness Training: The Proven Program for Raising Responsible Children*, Three Rivers Press.

Granju, K., (1999). *Attachment Parenting: Instinctive Care for Your Baby and Young Child*, Pocket Books.

Harper, B., (1994). *Gentle Birth Choices: A Guide to Making Informed Decisions about Birthing Centers, Birth Attendants, Waterbirth, Homebirth and Hospital Birth*, Healing Arts Press.

Karr-Morse & Wiley, (1977). *Ghosts from the Nursery: Tracing the Roots of Violence,* Atlantic Monthly Press.

Katz-Rothman, B., (1993). *The Tentative Pregnancy: How Amniocentesis Changes the Experience of Motherhood,* W.W. Norton & Co.

Liedloff, J., (1995). *The Continuum Concept; In Search of Happiness Lost,* Addison-Wesley Publishing Company.

Maushart, S., (2000). *The Mask of Motherhood: How Becoming a Mother Changes Our Lives and Why We Never Talk About It,* Penguin Books.

McGraw, P., (1999) *Life Strategies: Doing What Works, Doing What Matters.* Hyperion.

Ruiz, M., (1997). *The Four Agreements: A Practical Guide to Personal Freedom,* Amber-Allen.

Mongan, M., (1998). *HypnoBirthing®, A Celebration of Life: A Definitive Guide for Easier, Safer, More Comfortable Birthing,* Rivertree Publishing.

Northrup, C., (1998). *Women's Bodies, Women's Wisdom,* Bantam Books.

Pantly, E., (2002). *The No Cry Sleep Solution: Gentle Ways to Help Your Baby Sleep Through the Night,* Contemporary Books.

Pearce, J., (1977). *Magical Child,* Plume.

Robbins, J., (1996). *Reclaiming Our Health: Exploding the Medical Myth and Embracing the Source of Healing,* HJ Kramer.

Schlessinger, L., (2000). *Parenthood by Proxy: Don't Have Them If You Won't Raise Them,* HarperCollins.

Stewert, D., (1981). *The Five Safe Standards for Safe Childbearing,* NAPSAC Intl.

Strong, T., (2000). *Expecting Trouble: The Myth of Prenatal Care in America,* New York University Press.

Tamoro, J., (1995). *So That's What They're For!,* Adams Media Corp.

Wagner, M., (1994). *Pursuing the Birth Machine: The Search for Appropriate Birth Technology,* A.C.E. Graphics.

Wolf, N., (2001.) *MisConceptions: Truth, Lies and the Unexpected on the Journey to Motherhood,* Doubleday.

Williams, P., (2002). *The PTSD Workbook: Simple, Effective Ways for Overcoming Traumatic Stress Symptoms,* New Harbinger Publications, Inc.

Web Resources

Every attempt has been made to assure the resources listed below are current, but the internet is an ever changing medium. Please let the author know of any changes found that should be made in future editions.

Alliance for the Improvement of Maternity Services
http://www.aimsusa.org/

Breastfeeding Online, Dr. Jack Newman
http://www.breastfeedingonline.com/newman.shtml

Citizens for Midwifery
http://www.cfmidwifery.org/

Coalition for Improving Maternity Services
http://www.motherfriendly.org/

The Cochran Collaboration
http://www.cochrane.org/

Henci Goer Articles
http://www.hencigoer.com/articles/

The International Cesarean Awareness Network
http://www.ican-online.org/

Midwifery Today Online
http://www.midwiferytoday.com/

Mothering
http://www.mothering.com

NARM (North American Registry of Midwives)
www.narm.org

Safety and Cost Effectiveness of the Midwifery Model of Care
http://www.collegeofmidwives.org/collegeofmidwives.org/safety_issues
01/safetyIndex01.htm

Cesearan rates per hosptial or region:

CesareanRates.com
http://www.cesareanrates.com/blog/2012/8/17/did-tort-reform-in-texas-lower-the-states-total-cesarean-rat.html

WeBirth
http://www.ourrealvillage.com/cesareanlocal#michigan

The Birth Survey
http://thebirthsurvey.org/dev/Results/learn_state.shtml

Independent Childbirth Classes

The Association of Labor Assistants and Childbirth Educators
http://www.alace.org/education/

Birthing from Within
http://www.birthingfromwithin.com

The Bradley® Method of Husband Coached Childbirth
http://www.bradleybirth.com

Childbirth International
http://www.childbirthinternational.com

Lamaze® International
http://www.lamaze.org

The Original Mongan Method HypnoBirthing®
http://www.hypnobirthing.com/

Ultrasound Safety

Midwifery Today
http://www.midwiferytoday.com/articles/default.asp?a=1&r=1&e=1&q=ultrasound

Midwife Archives
http://www.gentlebirth.org/archives/preScreen.html

Cited Works

ACDE, (1999). American Council for Drug Education. *Basic Facts About Drugs*. Retrieved July 2, 2012 at
http://www.acde.org/common/Tobacco.htm

ADA, (2012). American Diabetes Association, Standards of Medical Care in Diabetes. *Detection and diagnosis of gestational diabetes mellitus (GDM)*. Retrieved July 9, 2012 from
http://care.diabetesjournals.org/content/35/Supplement_1/S11.full

Arms, S., (1994) *Immaculate Deception II: Myth, Magic and Birth*. Celestial Arts.

Association for Improvements in Maternity Services, (AIMS)
www.aims.org.uk
http://www.aimsusa.org/ObstetricDrugs-NotApproved.htm

Autims Today, (nd). *ATTN: Researchers-Look in the first environment, the womb*. Retrieved August 26, 2012 from
http://www.autismtoday.com/articles/ATTN_Researchers.htm

Ayers, S., Pickering, A., 2001. *Do Women Get Post-traumatic Stress Disorder as a Result of Childbirth? A prospective study of incidence*. Birth, 28 (2).

Beech, B., Robinson, J., 1994. *Ultrasound Unsound?* London: AIMS.

Blaffer Hrdy, S., (1999). *Mother Nature, A History of Mothers, Infants, and Natural Selection*. Pantheon Books.

Brown, D., Murphy, M., (1996). *Medical Hypnosis in Preterm Labor, A randomized Clinical Trial*.

Buchsbaum G., Chin M., Glantz C., Guzick D., (2002). *Prevalence of urinary incontinence and associated risk factors in a cohort of nuns*. Obstet. Gynecol. 2002 Aug;100(2):226-9. Retrieved February 2, 2012 from http://
www.ncbi.nlm.nih.gov/pubmed/12151141

CBS News, 2010. *More Breastfeeding Could Save 900 Lives a Year.* [Website News Article]. CBS News, April 5. Retrieved November 9, 2011 from: http://www.cbsnews.com/stories/2010/04/05/health/ main6364292.shtml

CDC, (2012). *Antibiotic/Antimicrobial Resistence.* Centers for Disease Control. Retreieved August 25, 2012 from http://www.cdc.gov/drugresistance/actionplan/taskforce.html

Central Intelligence Agency (CIA), 2011-Updated Weekly. *The World Factbook. Country Comparrisson: Infant Mortality Rate.* [Webpage]. Retrieved November 8, 2011 from: https://www.cia.gov/library/publications/the-world-factbook/rankorder/ 2091rank.html

Childbirth Connection, 2011. *Cesarean Section: Why does the National U.S. Cesarean Section Rate Keep Going Up?* [Webpage]. Retrieved September 14, 2011 from: http://www.childbirthconnection.org/article.asp?ck=10456

Childbirth.org, (1997). *Mode of Delivery for Breech Presentation.* [Web Resource]. Retrieved November 9, 2011 from: http://www.childbirth.org/section/vagbreech.html

Childbirth.org, (1998). *Amniotomy FAQs.* Retrieved August 28, 2012 from http://www.childbirth.org/articles/amnio.html).

CIA (2011). *CIA World Fact Book.* Retrieved July 2, 2012 from https://www.cia.gov/library/publications/the-world-factbook/rankorder/2091rank.html

CIMS, Current. Coalition for Improving Maternity Services. [Webpage]. Retrieved November 8, 2011 from: http://www.motherfriendly.org/MFCI/

Carr-Morse, R., Wiley, M., (1997). *Tracing the Roots of Violence.* Atlantic Monthly Press.

Davis-Floyd, R., (2004) *Birth as An American Rite of Passage, 2nd ed.* University of California Press.

Deirse, M., (1984). Bet-Mimetic Drugs in the Prophylaxis of Preterm Labour: Extent and   Rationale of Their Use. *British Journal of Obstetrics and Gynecology.* 91 (1984) 431

Ehrenthal, D., Xiaozhang J., Strobino, D. (2010). Labor Induction and the Risk of a Cesarean Delivery Among Nulliparous Women at Term. *Obstetrics & Gynecology;* Jul2010, Vol. 116 Issue 1, p35 42. Accessed July 9, 2012 via Academic Search   Premier.

Enkin M., Keirse M., Renfrew, M., Neilson, J., (1995). *A Guide to Effective Care in Pregnancy and Childbirth. 2nd ed.* Oxford University Press, Falco, R. (nd.) *Gentle Birth Midwife Archives.* Retrieved December 28, 2011 from   http://www.gentlebirth.org/archives/homsafty.html

FDA, (2009). Misoprostol (marketed as Cytotec) Information; *FDA ALERT – Risks of Use in Labor and Delivery. U.S. Food and Drug Administration.* Retrieved August 26, 2012 from http://www.fda.gov/Drugs/DrugSafety/ postmarketDrugSafetyInformationforPatientsandProviders/ ucm111315.htm

FDA, (2011). *Antibiotics and Antibiotic Resistance.* U.S. Food and Drug Administration. Retrieved August 25, 2012 from www.fda.gov/Drugs/ResourcesForYou/Consumers/BuyingUsingMedicin eSafely/AntibioticsandAntibioticResistance/default.htm

Frye, A., 1993. *Understanding Diagnostic Tests in the Childbearing Year. 5th ed.* Portland, OR: Labrys Press.

Goer, H., Midwifery Today, 2002. *The Assault on Normal Birth: The OB Disinformation Campaign.* [Archived article]. Retrieved November 8, 2011 from: http://midwiferytoday.com/articles/disinformation.asp

Graves, J., Miller, K., Sellers, A., (2002). Maternal Serum Triple Analyte Screening in Pregnancy. *Am Fam Physician.* 2002 Mar 1;65(5):915-921.

Greene, A., (2002). *Brain Size and ADHD.* Retrieved July 16, 2012 from http://www.drgreene.com/21_1016.html

Greve, P. (2009). *Labor Pains: Liability trends in obstetrics.* Liability Monitor. Retrieved July 3, 2012 from http://www.scpcf.com/PDF/MLM_LaborPains08_09.pdf

Guinn, D., Goepfert, A., Own, J., Wentrom, K., Hauth, J., (1988). Terbutaline Pump Maintenance Therapy for Prevention of Preterm Delivery: A Double-Blind Trial. *American Journal of Obstetrics and Gynecology.* 179(1998)874

Harmon, T., Hynan M., Tyre T., (1990). Improved obstetric outcomes using hypnotic analgesia and skill mastery combined with childbirth education. *J Consult Clin Psychol* 1990; 58:525-30.

Hughes, J. Ph.D. (n.d.) *The Safety of Home Birth,* retrieved December 28, 2011 from http://www.changesurfer.com/Hlth/homebirth.html

Schultz, S., Klonoff-Cohen, H., Wingard, D., Akshoomoff, N., Macera, C., Ji, M., & Bacher, C., (2006). Breastfeeding, infant formula supplementation, and Autistic Disorder: the results of a parent survey. *International Breastfeeding Journal.* Retrieved August 28, 2012 from http://www.internationalbreastfeedingjournal.com/content/1/1/16/

Karr, R., Wiley, M., 1997. *Ghosts from the Nursery: Tracing the Roots of Violence.* New York: Monthly Press.

Klaus, H., Kennell, J., Klaus, P., (1996). *Bonding: Building The Foundations Of Secure Attachment And Independence.* Da Capo Press.

Klaus, M., (1993). *Mothering The Mother: How A Doula Can Help You Have A Shorter, Easier, And Healthier Birth.* Da Capo Press.

Kotaska, A., Menticoglou. S., Gagnon, R., Farine, D., Basso, M., Bos, H., Delisle, M., Grabowska, K., Hudon, L., Mundle, W., Murphy-Kaulbeck, L., Ouellet, A., Pressey, T., Roggensack, A.; Maternal Fetal Medicine Committee; Society of Obstetricians and Gynaecologists of Canada. Vaginal delivery of breech presentation. J Obstet Gynaecol Can. 2009 Jun;31(6):557-66, 567-78.

Lazar, P., Gueguen, S., Dreyfus J., (1984). Multi-centered controlled trial of cervical cerclage in women at moderate risk of preterm delivery. *British Journal of Obstetrics and Gynaecology* 91(8).

Lenihan JP., (1984). Relationship of antepartum pelvic examinations to premature   rupture of the membranes. *Obstet Gynecol* 1984;63 (1):33-37

Liedloff, J., (1995). *The Continuum Concept.* Addison-Wesley Publishing.

Macones, G., Berlin, M., Berlin, J., (1977). Efficacy of Oral Beta-Agonist Maintenance Therapy in Preterm Labor: A Meta-Analysis. *Obstetrics and Bynecology.* 85(2001)313

Main, D., Main, E., (1986). Management of Preterm Labor and Delivery. *Obstetrics: Normal and Problem Pregnancies.* S.G. Grabbe, J.R. Hiebyl, J.L. Simpson, editors.   New York: Churchill Livingstone, 1986, p. 689

March of Dimes, 2009. March of Dimes Foundation Data Book for Policy Makers. Retrieved November 8, 2011 from http://www.rememberthemothers.net/

March of Dimes, (2009). *March of Dimes Foundation Data Book for Policy Makers: Maternal, Infant, and Child Health in the United States 2010.* http://www.marchofdimes.com/Databookforpolicymakers.pdf

March of Dimes, (2010). http://www.marchofdimes.com/baby/premature_indepth.html

Mayer, E., et al, 1988. Reduced Risk of IDDM Among Breastfed Children. *Diabetes,* (37), p. 1625-1632.

McDuffie RS et al. Effect of routine weekly cervical examinations at term on premature   rupture of the membranes; a randomized controlled trial. *Obtset Gynecol* 1992;79(2);219-222.

Medical News Service, (2003). *Doctor Issued Patent on Biomarker Linking Autism, ADD and ADHD.* Retrieved July 16, 2012 from www.medicalnewsservice.com/ARCHIVE/ MNS1585.cfm

Mehl, L. , 1994. Hypnosis and Conversion of the Breech to the Vertex Presentation. *Fam Med,* 3, p. 881-887.

Mirkin, G., 1999. *Breast Milk Prevents Childhood Diabetes?* [Website]. Retrieved November 9, 2011 from Breast milk prevents Childhood Diabetes, 1999, http://www.drmirkin.com/diabetes/D216.htm

Mona Lydon-Rochelle, Holt, V., Easterling, T., Martin, D., (2001). Risk of Uterine Rupture during Labor among Women with a Prior Cesarean Delivery. *New England Journal of Medicine*, Vl 345, No. 1, July 5, 2001. Retrieved July 9, 2012 from http://www.nejm.org/doi/pdf/10.1056/NEJM200107053450101

Morley, G. (nd) *Birth Injuries Related to Umbilical Cord Clamping.* Retrieved August 27, 2012 from http://www.cordclamp.org

Mothering Magazine, 2010. *Shocked at Epidural Rates!* [Web discussion]. Retrieved November 11, 2011 from: http://www.mothering.com/community/t/1201454/shocked-at-epidural-rates

NBC Nightly News with Tom Brokaw, (2002). *Some States Facing ob-gyn shortage.* May 8, 2002.

Null, G., 2009-2011. *Vaccines.* [Collection of Articles]. Retreived November 9, 2011 from: http://www.garynull.com/home/category/vaccines

NVIC, (2012). *Introduction to autism informatoin. National Vaccine Information Center.* Retrieved August 28, 2012 from http://www.nvic.org/vaccines-and-diseases/ Autism.aspx

Odent, M., (1999). *The Scientification of Love.* Free Association Books.

Pang J, Heffelfinger J, Huang G, Benedetti T, Weiss N., 2002. Outcomes of planned home births in Washington state: 1989-1996. *Obstet Gynecol*, 100(2):253-59.

Pearce, J., (1992). *Magical Child.* Plume Books.

Reinberg, S., 2011. C-section rate in U.S. climbs to all-time high. [Website]. USA Today; Your Life, July 22, 2011. Retrieved September 14, 2011 from: http://yourlife.usatoday.com/parenting-family/pregnancy/story/2011/07/C-section- rate-in-US-climbs-to-all-time-high/49607756/1

Robbins, J., (1996). *Reclaiming Our Health,* pg. 24.

Robison, J., (2012). Ultrasound and Autism — A Connection? Could ultrasound energy have an effect on the developing fetus? *Psychology Today.* Retrieved August 26, 2012 from http://www.psychologytoday.com/blog/my-life-aspergers/201205/ultrasound-and-autism-connection

Rubin, R., (2002). Feb-up Obstetricians Look For a Way Out, *USA Today,* July 1, 2002.

Saftlas, A., Lawson, H., Atrash, H., (n.d.) Pregnancy related morbidity. From data to action: CDC's public health surveillance for women, infants and children. *Reproductive Heath of Women.* Retrieved August 26, 2012 from http://www.cdc.gov/reproductivehealth/ProductsPubs/DatatoAction/pdf/rhow10.pdf

Sakala, C., Corry, M., 2008. Evidence-Based Maternity Care: What It Is and What It Can Achieve. [Webpage Document]. Retrieved November 11, 2011 from http://www.milbank.org/reports/0809MaternityCare/0809MaternityCare.html

Schauble, P., Werner, W., Rai, S., Martin A., (1998). Childbirth preparation through hypnosis: the hynpnoreflexogenous protocol. *Am J Clin Hypnosis* 1998; 40:273-83.

Sepkoski, Lester, Osthemimer & Brazelton, 1992. The Effects of Maternal Epidural on Neonatal Behavior During the First Month. *Dev. Med Child Neurol,* 34 (12), p. 1072-80.

Simkin, P. (nd). http://www.pennysimkin.com/

Singh G, (2010). Maternal Mortality in the United States, 1935-2007:
Substantial Racial/Ethnic, Socioeconomic, and Geographic Disparities
Persist. A 75th Anniversary Publication. Health Resources and Services
Administration, Maternal and Child Health Bureau. Rockville, Maryland:
U.S. Department of Health and Human   Services; 2010. Retrieved July 5, 2012
from http://www.hrsa.gov/ourstories/mchb75th/
mchb75maternalmortality.pdf

Smith, C., nd. *Breastfeeding and Allergies: Protection Now and for the Future.*
[Web Article]. Retrieved November 9, 2011 from:
http://www.breastfeed.com/benefits-of- breastfeeding/breastfeeding-
and-allergies

Stewart, D., 1981. *The Five Standards for Safe Childbearing.* NAPSAC
International, p. 222.

Strong, T., (2000). *Expecting Trouble: The Myth of Prenatal Care in America.*
New York University Press.

Tuohy PG, (2003). Soy infant formula and phytoestrogens. *J Paediatr Child
Health.* 2003 Aug;39(6):401-5. Abstract retrieved August 23, 2012 from
http://www.ncbi.nlm.nih.gov/pubmed/12919490

Tyson, P.,(2001). The Hippocratic Oath Today. NOVA. *PBS Online.* Both
versions of the oath are found at:
http://www.pbs.org/wgbh/nova/doctors/oath_classical.html

Vedam, S., Schummers, L., Fulton, C., 2011. HOME BIRTH: An annotated
guide to the literature . [PDF Webpage]. Retrieved November 8, 2011 from:
http://www.bcmidwives.com/files/Home%20Birth%20Annotated%20gui
de%20to%20the%20literature%20May%202011.pdf

Wainer, N., Estner, L., (1983). *Silent Knife: Cesarean Prevention and Vaginal
Birth after Cesarean (VBAC).* Praeger.

Wagner, M., (1999). Ultrasound: More Harm than Good? *Midwifery Today.*
Issue 50, Summer 1999. Retrieved July 9, 2012 from
http://www.midwiferytoday.com/   articles/ultrasoundwagner.asp

Wagner, M., 2000. Technology in Birth: First Do No Harm. [Web Article]. *Midwifery Today*. Retrieved November 11, 2011 from http://www.midwiferytoday.com/ articles/technologyinbirth.asp

Wagner, M., 2001. What Every Midwife Should Know About ACOG and VBAC: Critique of ACOG Practice Bulletin No. 5, July 1999. Vaginal Birth After Previous Cesarean Section. *Midwifery Today*. http://midwiferytoday.com/articles/acog.asp.

Weiss, R., (2010). The myth of the vaginal exam in pregnancy. *Peaceful Parenting*. Retrieved August 26, 2012 from http://www.drmomma.org/2010/04/myth-of- vaginal-exam-in-pregnancy.html

Wenstrom, K., Wener, P., Merrill, D., Neibyl, J., (1977). A Placebo-Controlled, Randomized Trial of the Terbutaline Pump for Prevention of Preterm Delivery. *American Journal of Perinatology*.

Wilson, B., Effken, J., Butler, R. (2012). The Relationship Between Cesarean Section and Labor Induction. *Journal of Nursing Scholarship*; 2010 2nd Quarter, Vol. 42 Issue 2, p130-138. Accessed July 9, 2012 via Academic Search Premier.

Wax JR, Lucas FL, Lamont M, Pinette MG, Cartin A, Blackstone J., 2010. Maternal and newborn outcomes in planned home birth vs planned hospital births: a metaanalysis. *Am J Obstet Gynecol*, 203:243.e1-8.

Index

FDA (U.S. Federal Drug Administration), 114, 128, 136-137, 252, 306, 311

Formula, 30, 55, 56, 57, 94, 149, 161, 178, 287, 288

Gestational diabetes, 50, 68, 236, 281Goer,

Goer, Henci, 29, 47, 69, 139, 298, 298

Guilt, 38, 52, 62, 67, 77, 79, 80, 81, 93, 105, 108, 158, 172, 196, 260, 269, 293, 296, 301

Harper, Barbara, 29

Hippocratic Oath, 307

Home birth, 39, 48, 49, 50, 62, 66, 91, 92, 93, 114, 121, 144, 151, 152, 161, 193, 198, 208, 213, 218, 228, 229, 246, 254-255, 257, 282, 283

HypnoBirthing, 65, 86, 152, 162, 203, 207, 208, 211, 213, 214, 215, 222, 255

Hypnosis, 115, 141, 152, 162, 201, 210, 211, 212, 258

Infant mortality, 20, 84, 85, 229

Lawsuits, 105, 119, 129, 190, 248, 265, 266, 268, 273

Madera County Hospital, 265

MOD (March of Dimes), 20, 134, 135, 137

Maternal mortality, 20, 155, 266

Midwife/Midwifery, 42, 85, 92, 101, 114, 119, 121, 134, 144, 149, 206, 227, 254, 260, 266, 267, 279, 282

Malpractice, 67,105, 125, 128, 131, 190, 254, 264, 265, 266, 303

Misoprostol, 136

Mother's milk, 36, 56, 155, 156, 158

NARM, 317

Natural birth, 20, 27, 32, 33, 35, 40, 41, 64, 66, 70, 89, 107, 127, 152, 153, 155, 163, 174, 175, 177, 184, 191, 206, 213, 246, 284, 290, 292, 298-300

Nutrition, 54, 56, 68, 121, 124, 137, 138, 144, 149, 155, 190, 195, 254

Obstetrician, 46, 48, 50, 67, 83, 89, 101, 105, 141, 178, 197, 231, 249, 264-268, 273

Painless birth, **65, 70, 109, 124, 125, 161, 186, 198, 203, 206, 208, 209, 210-213, 215, 260, 286, 298, 299, 304**

Pang Study, 49

Pitocin, 32, 115, 116, 136, 154, 202, 270, 272, 311, 213

Postpartum depression (PPD), 55, 56, 67, 269, 270

About the Author

Kim Wildner has been a childbirth professional since 1991. Her passion is birth. When she isn't writing, teaching or lecturing she reads about birth, keeping abreast of the current literature. She also creates birth art through sculpture and other mediums. She has attended births in both home and hospital settings, has studied midwifery in the States and abroad, and has served in every capacity from labor assistant to primary midwife.

Wildner has had work published in Midwifery Today and Special Delivery, the journal of ALACE, the Association of Labor Assistants and Childbirth Educators.

She and her husband of 27 years live in Wisconsin. They have one gently home-born daughter.

Non-birth related interests include spending time with her family, walking, reading, knitting, beading and counted cross-stitch. She no longer enjoys camping, but could someday if a spectacular motorhome is involved.